# *Eat*
# *Your Way*
# *Thin*

# *Eat Your Way Thin*

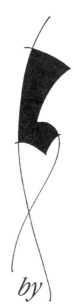

*by*

## Cynthia Martino
Nutritionist and Personal Trainer

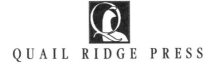

QUAIL RIDGE PRESS

# ACKNOWLEDGMENTS

Special thanks to Carolyn Winder who helped tremendously in developing low-fat versions of many of the delicious recipes contained within. Thanks also to my Mom, Aunt Pam, Cindy Martin, Judy Snyder and Anne Higgins for their contributions.

Library of Congress Cataloging-in-Publication Data

Martino, Cynthia.
    Eat Your Way Thin / by Martino, Cynthia.
        p.   cm.
    Includes index.
    ISBN 0-937552-76-3 (pbk.)
    1. Low-fat  diet--Recipes. 2. Reducing diets. I. Title.
RM237.7.M36   1996
641.5'638--dc21                               96-37197
                                                  CIP

**QUAIL RIDGE PRESS**
P. O. Box 123 · Brandon, MS  39043
1-800-343-1583

# CONTENTS

# ABOUT THE AUTHOR

Cynthia Martino has been in the diet and fitness "business" since she was four years old. Mrs. Martino was a gymnast at the young age of four, and competed until she was thirteen years old. At thirteen, Mrs. Martino spent three weeks training with the Romanian gymnastics team, along with Nadia Comaneci and a dozen gymnasts from the United States. Her gymnastic career was abruptly curtailed when she fractured a vertebra in her lower back.

Since her entire growing years were devoted to fitness and diet, Mrs. Martino focused her college education on nutrition and exercise physiology. Upon graduation, she began a personal training business in New York. For ten years, Mrs. Martino taught nutrition education courses in businesses and private schools, worked out with private clients, set up corporate fitness programs, and devoted her life to getting people in shape.

Mrs. Martino moved to Georgia in 1993, where she began a fitness training business, along with providing a low-fat cooking service for her clients. She wrote the book *Eat Your Way Thin* not only to teach people how to eat a balanced diet, but also to show how easy it is to prepare and cook delicious, low-calorie foods. The book provides dietary guidelines, a 30-day meal planner, and over a hundred sugar-free low-fat recipes. *Eat Your Way Thin* has been featured in *Atlanta Magazine* as well as the *Atlanta Business Chronicle.*

Mrs. Martino teaches a monthly low-fat cooking segment on Channel 11's *Noonday Program.* Additionally, she appears on WTLK TV-14, where she presents a half-hour talk show on diet, exercise, and low-fat cooking.

Mrs. Martino writes a weekly column for the *Forsyth County Newspaper* on healthy eating. She also writes a column for the Rolling Pin Kitchen Shop chain in their quarterly newsletter on healthy cooking techniques and recipe modification. Additionally, Mrs. Martino writes nutrition articles for the magazine *Women Looking Ahead.*

# INTRODUCTION

This low-calorie cookbook is designed for people who like to eat without having to worry about expanding their waistlines. Since I love to eat so much (and usually in large quantities), I have adapted the recipes so that they contain a large fiber content, and a very small fat content. My whole focus on eating, either for weight maintenance or weight loss, is to try to incorporate as many fruits and vegetables in the daily plan as possible. When you fill up on these low-calorie, high-fiber foods, you tend to eat less calories and fat overall.

All of the recipes are incorporated in a 1200-calorie diet plan. Each day is nutritionally balanced and focuses on balancing the proper quantity from each of the five food groups. The main emphasis is on carbohydrates, vegetables, and fruits. The daily plans are flexible, so that you can use the exchange list to substitute one food for another.

If your goal is to lose weight, I suggest you try the 1200-calorie diet plan. Additionally, exercise is an extremely important factor in losing weight and keeping it off. Any form of aerobic exercise, such as brisk walking, biking, running, aerobic dancing, or swimming is an excellent way to burn fat and increase your metabolism. Also, keeping a food diary will help you to lose weight and keep it off. The food diary makes you more conscious of what you put in your mouth, and helps to emphasize which food groups you may be lacking in or overindulging in. Studies have shown that one of the most influential factors in keeping the weight off is the continuation of writing daily intakes in a food journal. This just helps to reinforce good eating habits.

If your goal is to maintain your weight, use the cookbook to keep your diet low in fat. Although the daily food plans will be too low in calories for weight maintenance, you can still use them as a guideline towards consuming a high-carbohydrate, high-fiber diet.

Before initiating any dietary program, consult your

physician for a thorough physical examination. The dietary guidelines in this book are meant just for that purpose: to guide you towards a healthier life-style and way of cooking.

CM

# FOREWORD

In this age of fast-paced lifestyles, dual-income households, and cost-conscious consumption, we are all faced with the dilemma of satisfying one of our most fundamental requirements: eating properly. Although most of my patients and colleagues are aware of what constitutes a healthy, balanced diet, we often take the easy way out in terms of meal perparation. Ultimately, we all pay the price for our fast food appetites.

The majority of health problems treated today are self-inflicted by our own bad habits. The lack of adequate health maintenance and preventive health care is abundant in our society. If we treated our automobiles the way we treat our bodies, we'd all be walking to work—which may not be such a bad thing.

Fortunately, the interest in self-maintenance has become increasingly popular over the past decade, despite our stressful lifestyles. We now realize the serious long term implications of leading high stress, yet sedentary lives, coupled with poor dietary habits. The exercise book of the eighties provides mute testimony to the resurgence of interest in living healthier lives. In addition, recent medical research supporting the benefits of eating a balanced diet low in fat and cholesterol has provided us with ample justification for eating properly.

The recipes within this book have been carefully chosen to provide the reader with a healthy, balanced diet. The text has been cleverly designed as a meal plan which is based on the American Diabetic Association's diabetic exchange system. While calorie counting has been in vogue since the 1970s, the use of the diabetic exchange system has proven more useful in providing flexibility within the context of either weight loss or simply weight maintenance.

The value of this text can be measured in terms of its usefulness for not only losing weight safely, but keeping it off permanently by helping to structure healthier eating habits. The bonus to using this guide

9

is that the recipes are delicious. In fact, in some instances, it is difficult, if not impossible, to believe that some of the recipes are actually good for you. As an avid junk food aficionado who all too often catches my meals on the run, I can testify that the recipes described within this meal plan are both tasty as well as healthy . . . a rare combination.

Joseph A. Martino, M.D.
Orthopaedic Surgeon and
Sports Medicine Specialist

# HOW TO USE THE EXCHANGE LISTS

The exchange list breaks down food into six groups: **THE FRUIT GROUP, THE VEGETABLE GROUP, THE STARCH GROUP, THE PROTEIN GROUP, THE MILK GROUP**, and **THE FAT GROUP**. As you look at each food group, you will notice that every food item listed has a quantity after it. For example, in the fruit group, one apple (2-inch diameter) is equivalent to 1/3 cup of apple juice. This means that for the same amount of calories, you may get a larger quantity of certain fruits, in various forms, than others.

For instance, you could either have one small apple or one-half of a small banana. Try to choose foods that you can eat a larger quantity of, since this will make you feel more full and satisfied. When you bulk up on these high-fiber, low-calorie foods, you will tend to eat less of the higher calorie options. Therefore, your overall caloric intake will be less.

Based on the 1200-calorie diet plan, you will be allowed four from the Fruit group, four or more from the Vegetable group, six from the Starch group, four from the Protein group, two from the Milk group, and three from the Fat group. The protein content is probably much lower than you are used to eating, so you will have to plan ahead and use this towards your dinner meal most days. It will seem tricky initially, but with careful planning, it will become much easier.

**I. THE FRUIT GROUP**, from which you are allowed four exchanges, will help to get you through some of those between-meal munchies. Save a fruit for an in-between-meal snack, for instance before dinner or after dinner (or both) if those are your dangerous hours. It is always better to have the fresh fruit instead of juice, since it takes longer to eat, has more fiber in it, and will fill you up more. Also, dried fruits are higher in calories, since they are dehydrated and thus more concentrated. They are a fair source of iron, but you get less quantity for the same amount of calories. Try to include at least one fruit daily which is high in

Vitamin C, such as oranges, grapefruit, strawberries, and cantaloupe.

**II. THE VEGETABLE GROUP** is one of the biggest assets to any diet plan. Most vegetables, with the exception of the starchy ones, such as corn, peas, beans, etc., can be eaten in unlimited quantities. The more vegetables you add to your meal, the less your overall caloric consumption will be. Make your lunches more exciting and filling by adding as many vegetables to your sandwich as possible. Stuff pita bread with vegetables, and add low-fat cheese and dressing, or make vegetable tacos, and top them off with low-fat cheese and salsa. Emphasize vegetables at dinner, seasoning them with lemon pepper and other spices, and start the meal off with a fresh, crispy salad. Keep a bowl of cut-up, cleaned raw vegetables to snack on with some of your favorite low-calorie yogurt or cottage cheese dips as an in-between-meal snack.

**III. THE STARCH GROUP**, from which you may have six exchanges, should be the focus of your dietary plan. Try to have whole grain breads and cereals instead of the highly processed white flour variety. Check the nutritional panel on your favorite breads and cereals to determine the overall nutritional value and fat content. Certain types of bread, those containing nuts and seeds, are very high in fat. Try to select breads and rolls that are approximately 70 calories per ounce, which corresponds to the amount in each starch exchange on your list.

Portion size in ready-to-eat cereals is something else you should be leery of. For instance, one ounce of Grape Nuts cereal, which is approximately 1/4 cup, is about 100 calories. The caloric value of one ounce of Cheerios cereal is also approximately 100 calories, but the quantity is 1 1/4 cups. It is very important that you use a measuring cup to measure these, initially at least. Once you have seen what your portion size looks like in a bowl, you may eventually want to just eyeball the portion size.

Another important aspect to think about regarding the starch group is the size of bagels and muffins.

Lender's bagels, which are found in the freezer case, are considered two bread exchanges each. However, a large bagel from the grocery store or a Bruger's Bagel is considered three bread exchanges. If you plan on having a large bagel for breakfast, just remember that you have only three more bread exchanges for the rest of the day.

The same thing goes for muffins. Large muffins, such as blueberry bran, or corn, are considered three bread exchanges. Even worse, they are loaded with fat (from oil), and thus are very high in calories.

Another point to be discussed is the quantity of one exchange of pasta and rice in the starch group. One-half of a cup is considered one starch exchange. If you plan on going out for Italian food some night, you will have to save up four starch exchanges for two cups of pasta! Plan ahead!!

IV. The number of exchanges from **THE PROTEIN GROUP** is much lower than most people are used to, as I mentioned earlier. Most people tend to save up their protein exchanges for their evening meal, focusing on carbohydrates, milk, fruit, and vegetables during the day. (Notice that a chicken breast, which is approximately 3 ounces, is equivalent to 3 protein exchanges!)

Try to have fish and poultry whenever possible, and when ordering out, ask for sauces on the side. Also, opt for broiled or grilled instead of baked and fried foods. Always remove the skin from poultry, since this is a saturated fat. Additionally, choose low-fat types of cheese while doing your grocery shopping.

V. **THE MILK GROUP**, from which you should have two exchanges, is very important. Your bones are constantly changing, and it is important to keep them strong by constantly replenishing them with calcium. By getting enough calcium in your diet now, you can help to prevent osteoporosis (bone thinning) in later years. If you are lactose intolerant, or just dislike milk, try some of the new no-sugar, no-fat yogurts. Dannon makes many delicious non-fat, non-sugar yogurts in such flavors as vanilla, cappuccino and various fruit combinations. If this does not suit your tastes, you may want to take a calcium supplement. Look for calcium supplements that contain calcium carbonate (1200 mgs./day), since these are absorbed the best.

**VI. THE FAT GROUP**, from which you are allotted three exchanges, may be difficult to restrict. Be aware of just how small the portions are in each exchange. For instance, one teaspoon of butter is one fat exchange or forty calories. For that same forty calories, you could eat a small apple, which would be much more filling. When cooking, use a measuring spoon so that you can see how many fat calories you are adding to your food. Instead of using oil or butter to sauté, use nonstick pans sprayed with a light coating of Pam cooking spray. Sauté vegetables and poultry in chicken bouillon, and use puréed tomatoes to sauté garlic and onion (instead of oil) when preparing spaghetti sauce. Also, if you are baking quick breads, substitute applesauce for the oil in the recipe.

When going out to dinner, it is very difficult to regulate how much fat is added to your food. Ask to have your fish entrée broiled or grilled with very little butter or none. If the entrée has a sauce, ask for it on the side. Ask the waitress to put your salad dressing on the side as well. You are paying for the meal, so ask to have it prepared the way you want it.

Notice that wine and liquor are considered fat exchanges. Three and one-half ounces of dry white wine equals 4 1/2 fat exchanges! Even worse, 1 1/2 ounces of an 80-proof liquor equals 3 fat exchanges! A 12-ounce beer equals 1 bread and 1 fat exchange. Don't let these fat calories sneak up on you. Plan ahead and incorporate them in your diet ahead of time.

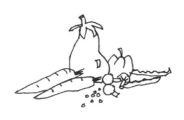

# HELPFUL HINTS

1. Think of your exchanges as an investment. If you want to have a 4-ounce piece of steak for dinner, plan on saving up your protein exchanges for the evening. You are allotted a certain amount from each food group—you get to decide how to spend them.

2. Plan ahead! It is much easier to follow a dietary plan if you decide on your meals for the week ahead of time. When cooking some of these low-calorie entrées, divide the meals into the portions suggested before serving your family. Freeze single portions, so that they can be pulled out, defrosted, and ready to serve for a last-minute dinner. If a recipe is supposed to make 10 portions, divide it into 10 servings immediately before your family has a chance to dig in. This allows you to control the portion size.

3. Do not skip meals. Even if you have a piece of fruit or a glass of milk in the morning, it is better than nothing. When you skip a meal, you tend to binge at the next, and set yourself up for lots of snacking.

4. Do not completely restrict yourself from foods you love. If you want to have pizza, for instance, just plan on using some of your fat, protein, and starch exchanges towards it. When you tell yourself, "I can't have that, I'm on a diet," you set yourself up for a binge. If you want a candy bar during the week as a treat, just plan on including it in your daily plan.

5. Try to eat meals at your kitchen table, without reading or watching television, or any other distractions. It is very easy to eat a bag of chips in front of the television, since you get so distracted by the program. All of a sudden you find that you have eaten an entire bag of chips, but you can't remember enjoying it that much. Reading while eating can have the same effect. You eat without realizing what and how much you are putting in your mouth.

**6.** Weigh yourself no more than once per week. Daily fluctuations with water weight can vary up to 5 pounds! Don't let yourself get discouraged by temporary water weight. An accurate reflection of fat loss can be seen by weighing yourself one day each week, in the morning before breakfast.

**7.** If you are going to a dinner party and plan to have a drink, look at the exchange value of the various alcoholic beverages. Three and one-half ounces of white wine equals 1 1/2 fats. If you want to invest your fat exchanges towards a drink, plan it into your diet.

**8.** If you do have a blow-out one day, it's not the end of the world. To make 1 pound of body fat, you need to eat 3500 calories over your normal daily intake. Think of your diet as a day-to-day mission. If you overeat one day, just get right back on your program the next. It's no big deal.

**9.** When you are getting ready to eat your next meal, take a minute to think about how long and how hard you would have to exercise to burn off the calories you are about to consume. For instance, if you wanted to have two scoops of ice cream as a treat, which contain approximately 300 calories, you would have to walk about one hour at a pace of 3.5 mph to burn it off!

I always ask myself, "Are those calories worth the effort to exercise them off?" Sometimes the answer is yes, but often I find that I am eating out of habit, boredom, or because I am tired. Look at the following chart to give you an idea about the calories burned during various activities. It sure is easier to put the calories in, than it is to burn them off!

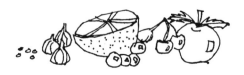

**Calories burned per hour:**

| Activity | 180 pounds | 130 pounds |
|---|---|---|
| Golf (Walking) | 410 | 299 |
| Tennis (Singles) | 520 | 375 |
| Tennis (Doubles) | 340 | 240 |
| Bicycling (10 mph) | 485 | 350 |
| Jogging (6 mph) | 755 | 545 |
| Rowing Machine | 555 | 400 |
| Swimming (slow crawl) | 630 | 450 |
| Walking (2 - 2.5 mph) | 385 | 305 |
| Walking (3.5 mph) | 430 | 310 |
| Weight Training | 340 | 245 |
| House Cleaning | 285 | 205 |

**10.** The fastest way to take the weight off and keep it off is by adding an exercise program to your low-fat eating plan. Aerobic exercise such as biking, running, brisk walking, and swimming, should be done at least three times per week. This type of exercise increases your metabolic rate, burning fat and many calories during the activity and, to a certain extent, for a few hours afterward. Strength training should be done at least three times per week as well. When you work on muscle-strengthening exercises in conjunction with dieting, a greater proportion of the weight loss will come from your fat stores than your muscles breaking down. This means that you conserve your muscle tissue, while breaking down the fat for energy. This is great news, because the more muscle you have, the higher your metabolic rate will be, and the more calories you will burn daily. The best exercise for you depends on what you enjoy doing. The fact is, if you do not like a specific exercise (ie. Step Aerobics), you will not keep it up. The most important thing to do is to find an activity you enjoy and keep on doing it! Make exercising a part of your day just as eating and sleeping are.

You didn't put the weight on overnight, so don't expect to lose it so quickly.

# THE EXCHANGE GROUPS

Based on a 1200-calorie diet plan, you will be allotted the following number of servings from each of the six food groups:

**4** from **The Fruit Group**
**4 or more** from **The Vegetable Group**
**6** from **The Starch Group**
**4** from **The Protein Group**
**2** from **The Milk Group**
**3** from **The Fat Group**

## THE FRUIT GROUP

Each portion below equals 1 serving of fruit and contains approximately 10 grams carbohydrate and 40 calories. You may have 4 servings from this group each day.

Apple (2" diameter)-1
Apple juice-1/3 cup
Apple sauce (unsweetened)-1/2 cup
Apricots (fresh)-1/2
Apricots (dried)-2 medium
Avocado-see fat exchange
Banana-1/2 small
Berries:
  Blackberries-1/2 cup
  Blueberries-1/2 cup
  Raspberries-1/2 cup
  Strawberries-3/4 cup
Cantaloupe-1/4 small
Cherries (sweet) 10 large
Cider-1/3 cup
Cranberry juice-1/4 cup
Dates-2
Figs (fresh or dried)-1
Grapefruit-1/2
Grapes:
  Large-12

Thompson seedless-1/2 cup
Grape juice-1/4 cup
Guava-2/3
Honeydew melon-1/4 small
Mango-1/2 small
Nectarine-1 medium
Orange-1 small
Orange juice-1/2 cup
Papaya-1/3 medium, 3/4 cup
Peach-1 medium
Pear-1 small
Persimmon-1/2 medium
Pineapple (unsweetened)-1/2 cup
Pineapple juice-1/3 cup
Plums-2 medium
Prune juice-1/4 cup
Raisins-2 tablespoons
Unsweetened canned fruit-1/2 cup
Watermelon-1 cup

## THE VEGETABLE GROUP

Each portion below equals 1 vegetable serving and contains approximately 5 grams carbohydrate, 2 grams protein, and 25 calories. You may have 4 servings from this group each day.

Artichokes-1 whole, base and end of leaves
Asparagus
Bean sprouts
Cabbage
Carrots
Cauliflower
Celery
Chicory
Chives
Cucumbers
Eggplant
Escarole
Greens:
  Beet greens
  Chard
  Collards
  Dandelion
  Kale
  Mustard greens
  Poke
  Spinach

Lettuce
Mushrooms
Okra
Parsley
Peas
Peppers, green and red
Pumpkin
Radishes
Rutabagas
Tomato sauce
Tomato catsup-2 tablespoons
Turnips
V-8 juice-2/3 cup
Winter squash
Rhubarb
Sauerkraut
String beans
Summer squash
Tomatoes
Tomato juice-1/2 cup
Watercress
Zucchini squash

## THE STARCH GROUP

Each portion below equals 1 serving of starch and contains approximately 5 grams carbohydrate, 2 grams protein, and 70 calories. You may have 6 servings from this group each day.

**Breads:**

Bagel-1/2 Lender's or 1/3 large type
Biscuit (2" diameter)-1 (plus 1 fat exchange)
Bread (white, wheat, rye, pumpernickel, raisin, French, Italian)-1 slice or 1 ounce
Breadcrumbs-3 tablespoons
Breadsticks (9" diameter)-4

Buns (hot dog, hamburger)-1/2
Cornbread (1 1/2" squares)-1
Cracked wheat (Bulghar)-2 tablespoons
Croutons-1/2 cup
Diet slice bread-2 slices or 1 ounce
English muffin-1/2
Melba toast-4 slices

Muffins (unsweetened, 2"
   diameter)-1
Pita bread (6" diameter)-1
Pita-1/2 large
Popovers-1
Rolls (2" diameter)-1

Tortillas (6" diameter)-1
Waffles (5" diameter)-1
   (plus 1 fat exchange)

## Cereals* & Flours:
Bran flakes-1/2 cup
Cheerios-3/4 cup
Cooked cereals-1/2 cup
Grape Nuts-3 tablespoons
Puffed cereals (unsweet-
   ened)-1 1/2 cups
Other ready-to-eat cereals
   (unsweetened)-2/3 cup

Wheat germ-3 tablespoons
   or 1 ounce
Pasta (spaghetti, macaroni,
   noodles-cooked)-1/2 cup
Rice (cooked)-1/2 cup
Flours (all-purpose, whole
   wheat, rye, cornmeal,
   cornstarch)-3 tablespoons

*Check the side panel of your favorite cereal box to see what the serving size is for 1 ounce. One ounce should contain approximately 70 calories.

## Crackers:
Animal-8
Arrowroot-3
Cheese tidbits-35 or 3/4 cup
Graham (2 1/2" square)-2
Mr. Phipps pretzel chips-12
Matzo (4x6" diameter)-1
Milk-2
Oyster-20
Pretzels (3" sticks)-25
Rice cakes-2

Ritz-7 (plus 1 fat exchange)
Saltines-6
Snack Wells reduced fat
   cheese crackers-12
Soda (2 1/2" square)-4
Triscuits-5 (plus 1 fat
   exchange)
Wheat thins-12 (plus 1 fat
   exchange)
Wasa-2

## Starchy Vegetables:
Beans, peas & lentils (dried
   and cooked)-1/2 cup
Beans, baked (without
   pork)-1/4 cup
Corn on the cob (4" long)-1
Parsnips-1/4 cup
Potatoes (white-baked or
   boiled, 2" diameter)-1

Potatoes (white, mashed)-
   1/2 cup
Pumpkin (canned)-1 cup
Squash (winter, acorn, or
   butternut)-1/2 cup
Sweet potatoes or yams-1/4
   cup

**Miscellaneous:**

Frozen yogurt, nonfat &
  sugarfree-1 small
Ice cream-1/2 cup (plus 2
  fat exchanges)
Popcorn, popped-3 cups
Potato or corn chips-15 (plus
  2 fat exchanges)

Pancake (5 1/2" diameter) -
  1 (plus 1 fat exchange)
Sponge cake-1 1/2" cube
Waffle ( 5 1/2" diameter)-1
  (plus 1 fat exchange)

## THE PROTEIN GROUP

Each portion below equals 1 serving of protein and
contains approximately 7 grams protein, 5 grams fat,
and 70 calories. You may have 4 servings from this
group each day.

Note: You may use more than 1 serving per meal.
The weights should be taken on cooked meats.

### Fish & Seafood:

Any fresh or frozen-1 ounce
Canned crabmeat, lobster,
  salmon, tuna, mackerel-
  1/4 cup
  Note: 1 whole can of
  tuna (packed in water)=3
  proteins

Clams, oysters, scallops,
  shrimp-1 ounce or 5
  medium
Sardines (drained)-4 small
Surimi (imitation crab)-1
  ounce

### Meat:

Unless otherwise specified, 1 ounce is equal to 1 slice
approximately 3 x 5 x 1/8-inch thick.

Beef (roasts, steaks,
  ground)-1 ounce*
Frankfurters-1 small (plus 1
  fat exchange)
Lamb-1 ounce or 1/4 cup,
  chopped
Lamb chops-1 ounce or 1/2
  small chop
Liver-1 ounce**

Pork-1 ounce
Pork chops-1 ounce or 1/2
  small chop
Ham-1 ounce
Sausage-2 small (plus 1 fat
  exchange)
Spareribs-1 ounce without
  fat or 3 medium
Veal-1 ounce

*Whenever you buy beef or pork, select the most lean
meat possible.
**Liver has one of the highest cholesterol contents of
any food.

## Cold Cuts:

Bologna-1 ounce or 1/8" slice (plus 1 fat exchange)

Liverwurst-1 ounce or 1/4" slice (plus 1 fat exchange)

Salami-1 ounce or 1/4" slice (plus 1 fat exchange)

Vienna Sausage-2 1/2 (plus 1 fat exchange)

## Poultry

Cornish hen, guinea hen, pheasant-1 ounce

Chicken-1 ounce (1/4 chicken is approximately 3 ounces, thus 1 chicken breast equals 3 protein exchanges)

Chicken liver-1 ounces or 1 medium

Turkey-1 ounce or 1/8-inch slice

Other poultry-(capon, duck, goose, etc.)-1 ounce

## Cheese:*

All hard varieties (Cheddar) -1 ounce, 1/8" slice or 1" cube (plus 1 fat exchange)

Feta-1 ounce

Light & Lively Cottage Cheese (1% fat)-1/2 cup

Mozzarella, cottage, farmer, hoop, pot, ricotta-1/4 cup (plus 1 fat exchange)

Parmesan, romano-1/4 cup (plus 1 fat exchange)

*When selecting cheese at the grocery store, always choose the low-fat variety, or even better, the no-fat variety.

## Miscellaneous:

Eggs-1 medium (plus 1/2 fat exchange)*

Canadian bacon-1 ounce (plus 1/2 fat exchange)

Dried beans & peas-1/2 cup (plus 1 bread group)

Peanut butter-2 tablespoons (plus 2 fat exchanges)

Pizza-1 slice (plus 1 bread & 1 fat exchange)

*All of the cholesterol and fat are found in the yolk of the egg. When cooking or when making scrambled eggs, use 1 egg plus 2 egg whites, instead of 2 whole eggs.

## THE MILK GROUP

Each portion below equals 1 serving of milk and contains approximately 12 grams carbohydrate, 8 grams protein, and 80 calories. You may have 2 servings from this group each day.

**Non-Fat Fortified Milk:**

Skim/nonfat milk-1 cup

Buttermilk-1 cup

Yogurt (plain, unflavored)-1 cup

Sugarfree, nonfat yogurt (Dannon)-1 cup

Powdered (nonfat) 1/3 cup

Canned evaporated skim milk, before liquid is added-1/2 cup*

*Evaporated skim milk is excellent in coffee, and can be substituted for cream. If you don't like milk, this may be a way to get your milk exchanges in.

**Lowfat Fortified Milk:**

1% milk-1 cup (plus 1/2 fat exchange)

2% milk-1 cup (plus 1 fat exchange)

Yogurt made with 2% milk-1 cup (plus 1 fat exchange)

**Whole Milk:**

Whole milk-1 cup (plus 2 fat exchanges)

Yogurt made from whole milk (plain)-1 cup (plus 2 fat exchanges.)

Canned evaporated whole milk-1/2 cup (plus 2 Fat exchanges.)

## THE FAT GROUP

Each portion below equals 1 serving of fat and contains approximately 5 grams fat and 45 calories. You may have 3 servings from this group each day.

Avocado (4" diameter)-1/8

Butter*-1 teaspoon

Bacon, crisp*-1 slice

Bacon fat*-1 teaspoon

Cream, light*-2 tablespoons

Cream, heavy*-1 tablespoon

Cream, half and half*-2 tablespoons

Cream, sour*-2 tablespoons

Cream cheese*-1 tablespoon

Margarine, regular-1 teaspoon (soft, tub, or stick)

Margarine, diet-1 tablespoon

Mayonnaise*-1 1/2 teaspoons

Mayonnaise, imitation-1 tablespoon

Oils and cooking fats-1 teaspoon

Olives-5 small

Salad dressings:
   Low calorie (less than 25 calories per tablespoon)-3 tablespoons
   French, Italian-1 tablespoon
   Mayonnaise type-2 teaspoons

Sauces (Bernaise, Hollandaise, Tartar)*-1 teaspoon

Sesame seeds-2 teaspoons

Sunflower seeds-2 teaspoons

Nuts:
    Almonds-7
    Brazil nuts-2
    Cashews-5
    Coconut, shredded*-1
        tablespoon

Peanuts:
    Spanish 20
    Virginia-10
    Pecans-5 halves
    Pistachio-15
    Walnuts-5 halves

*These foods all contain saturated fat, which is the most damaging to your arteries.

## FREE FOODS

These foods contain so few calories that they may be used without any limit.

Coffee
Tea
Sugar-free soda
Bouillon/consummé (fat
    free)
Lemon
Unsweetened gelatin
Unsweetened pickles
Mustard
Horseradish
Saccharin and other non-
    caloric sweeteners

Herbs
Spices
Extracts
Soy sauce
Vinegar
Vegetables (except the
    starchy vegetables)
Diet dressings with less
    than 10 calories per
    tablespoon

## COMBINATION FOODS

### Soups*:
1 cup serving:
Chicken noodle-1/2 starch
Clam chowder-1 starch, 1
    protein
Cream of mushroom-1/2

starch, 2 fat
Split pea with ham-1 & 1/2
    starch, 1 protein
Tomato-1 starch, 1/2 fat
Vegetable-1 starch

*This group includes canned soups prepared according to manufacturers' directions. Campbell's makes many low-fat varieties. Look for the Healthy Request sign on the label.

## FAST FOOD RESTAURANTS

Hamburger, small-2 bread, 2
    protein, 1 fat exchange
Hamburger, large-2 bread, 3
    protein, 2 fat exchanges
Cheeseburger, small-2 bread,
    3 protein, 2 fat exchanges

Cheeseburger, large-2 bread,
    4 protein, 3 fat exchanges
French Fries, small-2 bread,
    2 fat exchanges
Fish Sandwich-2 bread, 2
    protein, 2 fat exchanges

## ALCOHOLIC BEVERAGES*

**Beer:**

Ale, mild, 12 oz.-147 calories
Beer, 12 oz.-171 calories-1 bread & 1 fat exchange
Light beer, 12 oz.-96

**Wines:**

Champagne, 3 oz-80 calories
Dubonnet, 3 oz-96 calories
Muscatel, 3 oz-120 calories
Port, 3 oz-120 calories
Red wine (dry), 3 oz-69 calories
Sherry (domestic), 3 oz- 72 calories

Vermouth (dry), 3 oz-75 calories
Vermouth (sweet), 3 oz-140 calories
White wine (dry/12% alcohol), 3 1/2 oz-74 calories-1 1/2 fat exchanges

**Liqueurs & Cordials:**

Creme de Cacao, 1 ounce-100 calories
Creme de Menthe, 1 ounce-112 calories
Curacao, 1 ounce-100 calories

Drambuie, 1 ounce-110 calories
Tia Maria, 1 ounce-113 calories

**Spirits:** Bourbon, brandy, cognac, whiskey, gin, rye, rum, scotch, tequila & vodka: 1 ounce:

80 proof-67 calories (1 1/2 ounces=3 fat exchanges)
84 proof-70 calories
90 proof-75 calories

94 proof-78 calories
97 proof-81 calories
100 proof-83 calories

*Remember that calories coming from alcohol are considered empty calories—they provide no nutrients, while contributing an abundance of calories. If you know that you are going to have a drink with dinner, plan on saving some of your fat exchanges towards it. It's your choice; you are allowed a certain amount from each food group, and you get to decide how you want to use them.

Take your diet one day at a time. If you overindulge one day, don't feel guilty and disgusted with yourself; just start right back the next day.

Some days you might want to increase the amount of calories that you are consuming. The following chart will show you how many exchanges you may have from each food group, while enjoying a balanced diet.

| Calories | 1200 | 1300 | 1500 | 1800 |
|---|---|---|---|---|
| Milk Group | 2 | 2 | 2 | 2 |
| Vegetable Group | 4-5 | 6 | 6-7 | 7-8 |
| Fruit Group | 4 | 5 | 6 | 7 |
| Carbohydrate/ Bread Group | 6 | 7 | 8 | 9 |
| Protein/Meat Group | 4 | 5 | 5 | 6 |
| Fat Group | 3 | 4 | 5 | 7 |

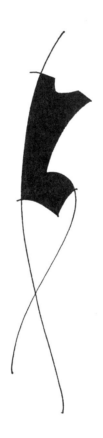

# FOOD DIARY

Every day you should keep a detailed list of what you have eaten. Try to write in it during the day or at the end of each day, since it is difficult to remember a day later exactly what you ate the day before. Make sure to measure portion sizes and be as accurate as you can. The food log that is provided below is a good template to use daily. Each line following the food group indicates a food exchange. For example, the Fruit Group has four lines after it, since you are allowed four exchanges from it. Fill the lines in as you use up your food exchanges from each food group during the day.

**4 Fruits:** _____
_____
_____
_____

**4 or More**
**Vegetables:** _____
_____
_____
_____

**6 Starches:** _____
(bread, pasta, rice, _____
crackers, corn, _____
peas, etc.) _____
_____
_____

**4 Proteins:** _____
(chicken, fish, _____
cheese, etc.) _____
_____

**2 Milks:** _____
_____

**3 Fats:** _____
(butter, oil, nuts, _____
seeds, etc.) _____

**4 Fruits:**

_____
_____
_____
_____


**4 or More Vegetables:**

_____
_____
_____
_____


**6 Starches:**
(bread, pasta, rice,
crackers, corn,
peas, etc.)

_____
_____
_____
_____
_____
_____


**4 Proteins:**
(chicken, fish,
cheese, etc.)

_____
_____
_____
_____


**2 Milks:**

_____
_____


**3 Fats:**
(butter, oil, nuts,
seeds, etc.)

_____
_____
_____

**4 Fruits:** _____
_____
_____
_____


**4 or More Vegetables:** _____
_____
_____
_____


**6 Starches:**
(bread, pasta, rice, crackers, corn, peas, etc.)
_____
_____
_____
_____
_____
_____


**4 Proteins:**
(chicken, fish, cheese, etc.)
_____
_____
_____
_____


**2 Milks:** _____
_____


**3 Fats:**
(butter, oil, nuts, seeds, etc.)
_____
_____
_____

**4 Fruits:**

_____
_____
_____
_____


**4 or More
Vegetables:**

_____
_____
_____
_____


**6 Starches:**
(bread, pasta, rice,
crackers, corn,
peas, etc.)

_____
_____
_____
_____
_____
_____


**4 Proteins:**
(chicken, fish,
cheese, etc.)

_____
_____
_____
_____


**2 Milks:**

_____
_____


**3 Fats:**
(butter, oil, nuts,
seeds, etc.)

_____
_____
_____

**4 Fruits:**

_____
_____
_____
_____


**4 or More
Vegetables:**

_____
_____
_____
_____


**6 Starches:**
(bread, pasta, rice,
crackers, corn,
peas, etc.)

_____
_____
_____
_____
_____


**4 Proteins:**
(chicken, fish,
cheese, etc.)

_____
_____
_____
_____


**2 Milks:**

_____
_____


**3 Fats:**
(butter, oil, nuts,
seeds, etc.)

_____
_____
_____

**4 Fruits:** _____
_____
_____
_____

**4 or More
Vegetables:** _____
_____
_____
_____

**6 Starches:**
(bread, pasta, rice,
crackers, corn,
peas, etc.)
_____
_____
_____
_____
_____
_____

**4 Proteins:**
(chicken, fish,
cheese, etc.)
_____
_____
_____
_____

**2 Milks:** _____
_____

**3 Fats:**
(butter, oil, nuts,
seeds, etc.)
_____
_____
_____

# Low-Fat Diet Plan for Day 1

*Breakfast:*
3/4 cup skim milk
2 ounces bran flakes
2 tablespoons raisins

*Lunch:*
Fruit Pita*

*Dinner:*
Fish with Salsa*
1 cup Spanish Rice *
1 cup skim milk

*Indicates recipe is provided below.


## FRUIT PITA

*Makes 1 serving.*
*1 serving = 3 Fruit, 2 Bread, 2 Fat, 1/4 Milk, 1 Protein*
    *Exchange.*
*430 calories per serving.*

1 large red delicious apple, finely chopped
12 grapes
1 ounce low-fat Cheddar cheese
1 whole wheat pita bread
1 cup shredded lettuce


## DRESSING:

1/4 cup plain nonfat yogurt
2 tablespoons apple sauce
1 tablespoon lime juice
1 tablespoon low-calorie light mayonnaise
1/4 teaspoon whole dried tarragon

Mix together the apple, grapes, and cheese.  Set aside.
Combine the dressing ingredients, and mix well with the
apple mixture until well coated.  Stuff the whole wheat
pita with the fruit, and garnish with the shredded lettuce.

# FISH WITH SALSA

*Makes 4 servings.*
*1 serving = 4 Proteins and 1 Vegetable Exchange.*
*280 calories per serving.*

1 pound fish (Any type of white fish like: flounder, sea
 bass, etc.)
2 cups salsa

Marinate the fish with your favorite salsa for at least 4
hours before cooking.

 Preheat oven to 350°. Place the fish on a nonstick baking sheet and top with the salsa used for marinating.
Cook for approximately 40 minutes, depending on the
type and thickness of fish. Garnish with fresh cilantro
if desired.

*Preparation Time: 5 minutes to prepare*
*Marinating Time: 4 hours*
*Cooking Time: 40 minutes*


# SPANISH RICE

*Makes 6 servings.*
*1 serving or 1/2 cup = 1 Bread and 1/2 Vegetable Ex-*
 *change.*
*80 calories per serving.*

3 cups precooked, cold rice
1/2 cup onion, chopped
1/4 cup bell pepper, chopped
1/2 teaspoon chili powder
1/2 teaspoon salt
3 teaspoons tomato paste
1 (14 1/2-ounce) can whole tomatoes, drained and chopped

In a nonstick skillet, sauté onions and bell pepper until
soft. Add tomatoes and cook for about 5 minutes. Add
the rice, chili powder, salt, and tomato paste. Serve immediately.

 **Note:** You may want to double the recipe, so that you
can use the remaining half for the diet plan the next
night.

*Preparation Time: 10 minutes*

# Low-Fat Diet Plan for Day 2

*Breakfast:*
1/2 English muffin with 1 tablespoon Polander All
    Fruit
1 cup skim milk
1 orange

*Lunch:*
Dagwood Sandwich
1 cup skim milk

*Snack:*
1 large apple

*Dinner:*
Chicken & Peppers*
1 1/2 cups rice
Large green salad with low-calorie dressing

**Note:** Save half of the Chicken & Peppers to have with
pasta on Day 3 of the diet.


## CHICKEN & PEPPERS WITH RICE
*Makes 4 servings.*
*1 serving = 4 Protein, 4 Bread, and 4 Vegetable Ex-*
    *changes.*
*570 calories per serving.*

2 pounds boneless chicken breast, cubed (visible fat
    removed)
Salt
Pepper
Cayenne pepper
3 large red bell peppers, cut in large pieces
3 large green bell peppers, cut in large pieces
2 medium white or yellow onions, cut in large pieces
1 small package fresh mushrooms, sliced (optional)
4 cups cooked rice (about 3 cups dry)

Season chicken with the salt, pepper, and cayenne to taste.
Place chicken in a nonstick skillet and brown. Add all
the vegetables and cook until the chicken is cooked thor-

*Continued*

oughly—approximately 35 minutes.  If desired, add more seasoning (salt, pepper and cayenne) to taste.

Serve over hot rice.

*Preparation Time:  30 minutes*
*Cooking Time:  35 minutes*


# DAGWOOD SANDWICH

*1 sandwich or 1 serving = 2 Bread, 1 Fat, 1 Protein, and 5*
  *Vegetable Exchanges.*
*300 calories per sandwich.*

2 slices whole wheat bread
1 tablespoon Miracle Whip Light
1 tablespoon yellow mustard
7 cucumber slices
1 ounce oven-roasted, sliced turkey breast
1/4 head of iceberg lettuce
2  slices tomato
1 large carrot, shredded
1/2 cup alfalfa sprouts
4 fresh mushrooms, cleaned and sliced (optional)
Cayenne pepper (optional)

Lightly toast the bread and spread with the Miracle Whip and mustard.  Place the cucumber slices, the turkey, the lettuce, tomato, shredded carrot, and sprouts (and mushrooms if desired) on the bread.  Sprinkle with cayenne. Press down firmly since all of the vegetables will make it difficult to fit in your mouth!  Remember, the more vegetables you load on the sandwich, the better.

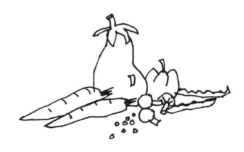

# Low-Fat Diet Plan for Day 3

*Breakfast:*
2 ounces cereal of your choice (Check the side panel
  to see what a 1-ounce serving size is.)
1 cup skim milk
1 small apple

*Lunch:*
Potato Skins (1 potato)*
Broccoli Salad*
1 cup skim milk

*Snack:*
24 grapes (Delicious when eaten frozen.)

*Dinner:*
1 serving Chicken & Peppers Over Pasta*
Large green leaf salad with tomato and low-calorie
  dressing

## POTATO SKINS
*1 potato skin from 1 whole potato = 1 Bread Exchange.*
*70 calories per potato skin.*

**4 large baking potatoes**
**Pam cooking spray**
**Salt and pepper to taste**

Preheat oven to 375°. Clean and wash the potatoes. Prick
with a knife, to allow the steam to escape, and bake 1
hour. Remove the baked potatoes and cut in half, scrap-
ing out the inside. Spray skins with cooking spray, season with the salt and pepper, and cook 15 minutes longer.

  These crispy skins may be used instead of bread at any
meal. Fill with tomato sauce and low-fat cheese for a
pizza potato, or stuff with your favorite vegetables and
top with low-fat sour cream, low-fat cheese or low-calorie salad dressing. (If you want to cook extras for another day, place in ziplock freezer bags and store in your
freezer until you are ready to use them.)

*Preparation: 5 minutes*
*Cooking Time: 1 hour 15 minutes*

# BROCCOLI SALAD

*Makes 5 servings.*
*1 serving  = 1 Vegetable, 1/2 Fruit, and 1/4 Protein*
  *Exchange.*
*40 calories per serving.*

1 pound fresh broccoli flowerets (1 bunch)
1/4 cup raisins
1 tablespoon bacon bits
1/2 cup Light & Lively low-fat (1%) cottage cheese,
  creamed in a blender
2 tablespoons chopped red onion
3 packets Sweet & Low
2 tablespoons white vinegar
1 tablespoon prepared mustard (dry spice)
1 clove garlic, minced

Wash and cut the broccoli, reserving the flowerets (discard stems).  Combine the broccoli, raisins, and bacon
bits.  Set aside.  Mix the cottage cheese, and the remaining ingredients, and toss together with the broccoli mixture.  May be served immediately.

*Preparation Time:  20 minutes*


# CHICKEN & PEPPERS OVER PASTA

*Makes 4 servings.*
*1 serving = 4 Protein, 1/4 Fat, 4 Bread, and 4 Vegetable*
  *Exchanges.*
*580 calories per serving.*

Chicken & Peppers (Reserved from night before if you
  doubled the recipe—See Index.)
1 (15-ounce) package prepared marinara sauce—Di Giorgno
  sauce is excellent!
4 cups cooked vermicelli (8 ounces dry)

Follow the recipe for Chicken & Peppers from the day
before, or use the leftover reserved from the night before
(if you doubled the recipe).  Mix all ingredients and enjoy.

*Preparation Time:  5 minutes*
*Cooking Time:  10 minutes*

# Low-Fat Diet Plan for Day 4

*Breakfast:*
2 Blueberry Bran Muffins*
1 cup skim milk

*Lunch:*
2 tortillas (6-inch diameter) with grilled vegetables
    (green peppers, red peppers, onion, mushrooms
    etc.), salsa, tomato, and shredded lettuce
1/2 cup skim milk

*Dinner:*
Oven-Fried Shrimp*
Mashed Potatoes*
Broccoli Salad* (See Index.)


## BLUEBERRY BRAN MUFFINS

*Makes 10 servings.*
*1 serving or 1 muffin = 1 Bread, 1/4 Fruit, and 1/4 Milk*
    *Exchange.*
*100 calories per muffin.*

2 cups Fiber One Cereal (General Mills), finely crushed
2 egg whites
1 1/2 cups skim milk
2 tablespoons applesauce
1 cup all-purpose flour
9 packets Sweet & Low
2 teaspoons baking powder
1/2 teaspoon baking soda
1/2 teaspoon salt
1 cup frozen blueberries, thawed, rinsed and drained

Preheat oven to 350°. Crush the cereal in a food processor. Mix the egg whites, milk, and applesauce. Mix all dry ingredients together. Add dry ingredients, including the cereal, to the egg mixture. Fold in blueberries. Spray nonstick muffin pans with Pam. Fill the muffin pans to the top and bake for 18 minutes or until toothpick inserted comes out clean.

*Preparation Time: 20 minutes*
*Cooking Time: 18 minutes*

# OVEN-FRIED SHRIMP

*Makes 4 servings.*
*1 serving = 4 Protein and 1/4 Fat Exchanges.*
*290 calories per serving.*

1 pound shrimp
Salt
Pepper
Cayenne
1 cup yellow cornmeal

Peel, devein, and butterfly the shrimp. Season with the salt, pepper, and cayenne to taste. Batter the shrimp in cornmeal only, and place on a nonstick pan.

Bake at 450° (on second rack from the top) for 25 minutes until golden brown.

*Preparation Time: 15 minutes*
*Cooking Time: 25 minutes*


# MASHED POTATOES

*Makes 2 servings.*
*1 serving = 2 Bread and 1/4 Milk Exchanges.*
*160 calories per serving.*

2 large baking potatoes
1/2 cup skim milk
1 teaspoon salt
Pepper to taste
1/2 tablespoon margarine

Preheat the oven to 400°. Scrub the potatoes and wrap them in foil. Place in the oven for 1 hour. Remove the foil and place the potatoes in a mixing bowl (with the skin on) and add warm skim milk and the rest of the ingredients. Mix with electric mixer until smooth.

**Note:** Adding a roasted garlic pod to the dish is a great option. (See Roasted Garlic in Index.)

*Preparation Time: 10 minutes*
*Cooking Time: 1 hour*

# Low-Fat Diet Plan for Day 5

*Breakfast:*
1 small Lender's Bagel
1 ounce low-fat cream cheese
1 cup skim milk
1 small banana

*Lunch:*
Vegetable Omelet*
English muffin
1 cup skim milk

*Dinner:*
Eggplant Parmesan*
Tomato with Ricotta*

*Snack:*
1 sugar-free fudgsicle

## VEGETABLE OMELET
*1 serving = 2 1/2 Protein and 4 Vegetable Exchanges.*
*215 calories per serving.*

1 egg and 2 egg whites
2 tablespoons low-fat milk
Salt and pepper to taste
1/2 green pepper, diced
1/2 red pepper, diced
1/4 onion, sliced thin
6 mushrooms, cleaned and sliced
1/2 tomato, sliced thin
1 ounce low-fat cheese (Feta, Mozzarella, etc.)

Combine the whole egg, egg whites, milk, and salt and pepper. Set aside. In a large nonstick skillet, sprayed with cooking spray, sauté the vegetables over a medium/ high heat until tender. Add a few tablespoons of water if the vegetables start to stick. When the vegetables have become tender (about 7 minutes), remove them from the heat. Set aside.

Over medium heat, place the milk mixture in a non-

*continued*

stick skillet and cook slowly. As the mixture starts to set, lift the egg from the side of the pan, allowing the uncooked egg on the top to run over onto the hot skillet. Add the vegetables and low-fat cheese; cook covered on low heat for 1 minute. Fold the egg mixture in half, covering the vegetable mixture, and serve immediately.

*Preparation Time: 15 minutes*
*Cooking Time: 10 minutes*


## EGGPLANT PARMESAN

*Makes 6 servings.*
*1 serving = 1 1/2 Protein, 1 Bread, 1 1/2 Fat and 2 Vegetable Exchanges.*
*255 calories per serving.*

2 small eggplants, cut in 1/4-inch slices
1/2 cup low-fat milk
1 package of mushrooms, sliced
1 jar tomato sauce (low-fat), or use the Sun-Dried Tomato Sauce* (See Index.)
1 cup (4 ounces) part-skim Mozzarella cheese

### BREAD CRUMB COATING:

1 cup bread crumbs
2 teaspoons basil
1 teaspoon Italian seasoning
1/2 teaspoon lemon pepper
1 teaspoon garlic powder
Red cayenne pepper, to taste

Cut eggplant and dip in milk wash, then into bread crumb mix. Place on cookie tray, and cook for 20 minutes at 425° until browned and crisped. Spray casserole dish with Pam and make a layer of eggplant, then mushrooms, then sauce. Layer again with eggplant, then mushrooms, then sauce, and top with Mozzarella cheese. Bake 350° for 40 minutes.

*Preparation Time: 30 minutes*
*Cooking Time: 40 minutes*

## TOMATO WITH RICOTTA

*1 serving = 1 Vegetable and 1/2 Fat Exchange.*
*25 calories per serving.*

2 cups green leaf lettuce
1 large tomato, sliced thick
1 1/2 tablespoons balsamic vinegar
1 tablespoon Ricotta cheese (low-fat)
Basil (preferably fresh)

Place bed of lettuce on salad plate. Add sliced tomato.
Pour the vinegar over the tomato and top with 1 tablespoon Ricotta cheese. Garnish with fresh basil.

*Preparation Time: 5 minutes*

Make your own low-fat salad dressings. Use 1 teaspoon each of
lemon pepper, garlic powder, dehydrated chives, Italian seasonings, and 2 packets of Equal, plus 1 teaspoon extra virgin
olive oil, and 3 tablespoons Balsamic vinegar.

---

# Low-Fat Diet Plan for Day 6

*Breakfast:*
1 cup skim milk
1 ounce oatmeal
1/2 small banana
3 tablespoons raisins

*Lunch:*
Pita bread, whole wheat
Spinach Salad with Apples & Raisins*

*Dinner:*
Jambalaya*
Green Beans with Carmelized Onions*
1 cup skim milk
1 (2-ounce) wheat roll

# SPINACH SALAD
# WITH APPLES & RAISINS
*1 serving = 4 Vegetable and 1 1/2 Fruit Exchanges.*
*80 calories per serving.*

1/2 teaspoon cinnamon
1/4 cup non-fat yogurt
1 packet Sweet & Low
2 cups fresh spinach
1 small apple, sliced
1 tablespoon raisins

Combine the cinnamon, yogurt, and Sweet & Low.   Mix
together the spinach, apple, and raisins; and toss with
the dressing.
   **Note:**  This is delicious when stuffed in a pita pocket.

*Preparation Time: 15 minutes*


# JAMBALAYA
*Makes 5 servings.*
*1 serving = 4 Protein, 1/4 Fat, 1 1/4 Vegetable, and  1*
   *Bread Exchanges.*
*390 calories per serving.*

3/4 pound turkey sausage sprinkled with salt, red pepper,
   and black pepper
1/2 cup bell pepper, chopped
8 ounces chicken
3 cups raw shrimp (optional)
3 (16-ounce) cans of whole tomatoes, drained and puréed
2 1/2 cups water
1 large onion, chopped
2 tablespoons parsley
2 cups raw rice
1 1/4 teaspoons salt
2 tablespoons Worcestershire
1/2 teaspoon thyme
1/4 teaspoon red pepper

Prepare turkey sausage in a nonstick pan.  Sprinkle 1 side
with salt, red pepper, and black pepper; sear seasonings
onto sausage.  Turn over and sprinkle the other side with
only red pepper.  Set aside.

*continued*

Sauté the bell pepper for 5 minutes in a large Dutch oven. Add meats, tomatoes, water, onions, garlic, and parsley. Bring to a boil, then add rice, salt, Worcestershire, thyme, and red pepper. Cover and simmer until rice is tender and liquid is absorbed. Add more seasonings to taste, if desired.

*Preparation Time: 20 minutes*
*Cooking Time: 45 minutes*


# GREEN BEANS
# WITH CARAMELIZED ONION

*Makes 4 servings.*
*Free vegetable.*

1 1/2 pounds fresh green beans
1 medium onion
Salt, pepper, and cayenne to taste

Snap and wash the beans. Chop the onion and cook slowly in a nonstick pan until they are a caramel color. (Add some water if the onion starts to stick.) Add the beans, add 1/2 inch water to pan, and cover. Steam beans until cooked, but still firm. Add seasoning and stir.

*Preparation Time: 20 minutes*
*Cooking Time: 35 minutes*

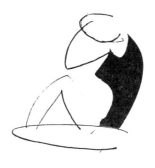

# Low-Fat Diet Plan for Day 7

*Breakfast :*
2  Pineapple-Carrot Muffins*
1 cup skim milk

*Lunch:*
Vegetable Pocket
1 cup skim milk

*Snack:*
1 large orange

*Dinner:*
Chicken Breast Dijon*
Pasta Primavera*  (Save some for next day's lunch.)

## PINEAPPLE—CARROT  MUFFINS
*Makes 10 muffins.*
*1 serving or 1 muffin = 1/4 Fruit,  1 Bread, and 1/4 Milk Exchange.*
*100 calories per serving.*

2 cups Fiber One Cereal (General Mills), finely crushed
2 egg whites
1 1/2 cups skim milk
2 tablespoons applesauce
1 cup all-purpose flour
6 packets Sweet & Low
2 teaspoons baking powder
1/2 teaspoon baking soda
1/2 teaspoon salt
3/4 cup crushed pineapple, drained
1/2 cup grated carrots

Preheat oven to 350°. Crush cereal in food processor. Mix egg, milk, and applesauce.  Mix all dry ingredients together.  Add dry ingredients, including the cereal, and the egg mixture. Fold in the pineapple and carrots. Spray nonstick muffin tins with Pam, and fill the tins to the top with the batter.  Cook approximately 25 minutes or until toothpick inserted comes out clean.

*Preparation Time:  20 minutes*
*Cooking Time:  25 minutes*

# CHICKEN BREAST DIJON

*Makes 4 servings.*
*1 serving or 1 chicken breast = 4 1/4 Protein, 1/2 Fat,*
  *and 1/2 Bread Exchange.*
*355 calories per serving.*

4 (4-ounce) chicken breasts, skinned and boned
1 tablespoon Miracle Whip Light
1 tablespoon mustard
1/2 teaspoon thyme
Pepper, to taste
1/3 cup bread crumbs
1 tablespoon Parmesan cheese

Preheat oven to 375°. Brush chicken with a mixture of the Miracle Whip, mustard, thyme, and pepper, then dredge in bread crumbs and Parmesan mixed. Place on a cookie sheet sprayed with Pam, and bake 45 minutes.

*Preparation Time: 15 minutes*
*Cooking Time: 45 minutes*

# PASTA PRIMAVERA

*Makes 10 servings.*
*1 serving or 1 cup = 2 Bread and 1/2 Vegetable Exchange.*
*150 calories per serving.*

1 pound tricolor pasta spirals (8 cups dry = 10 cups cooked)
2 large red peppers, diced
2 large green peppers, diced
1/2 large red onion, diced
1/2 cup fat-free Italian dressing (Ken's Light Caesar is
  terrific!)
1 tablespoon basil
1 teaspoon mustard (optional)

Bring a large pot of water to a boil and cook the pasta al dente. Drain it in a colander and run cold water over it to prevent further cooking.

Mix together the dressing, basil, and mustard, and combine with the pasta and vegetable mixture.

**Note:** This is delicious with Feta cheese.

*Preparation Time: 20 minutes*
*Cooking Time: 8 minutes*

# Low-Fat Diet Plan for Day 8

**Breakfast:**
Nonfat, sugar-free Dannon Yogurt—any flavor
1 cup blueberries or canned unsweetened fruit

**Lunch:**
1 cup Pasta Primavera* (Left over from the previous
    night. See Index.)
2 ounces Surimi (imitation crab)
1 cup skim milk

**Snack:**
1 small banana

**Dinner:**
1 cup lentils*
1 cup rice
Marinated Tomato Salad*

## LENTILS
*1 serving or 1/2 cup = 1 Bread Exchange.*
*70 calories per serving.*

**1 package lentils**
**1 large onion**
**1 large bell pepper**
**3 bay leaves**
**1 tablespoon salt**
**1 tablespoon cayenne**
**1 teaspoon black pepper**

Rinse lentils and drain. Chop onion and bell pepper, and
sauté in water until tender. Add lentils and water, 1 inch
above the beans, and the rest of the seasonings. Cover
and cook 2 1/2 hours. Adjust seasoning to taste.

*Preparation Time: 10 minutes*
*Cooking Time: 2 1/2 hours*

# MARINATED TOMATO SALAD

*Makes 6 servings.*
*1 serving = 1 Vegetable Exchange.*
*20 calories per serving.*

8 large tomatoes
3/4 cup red wine vinegar
5 cloves garlic, crushed
2 teaspoons salt
1 teaspoon freshly ground black pepper
1/2 cup fresh basil (if basil isn't available, use spinach
    leaves)
4 ounces Feta cheese (optional)—If you haven't used all
    your Protein Exchanges, include the Feta cheese. It's
    delicious!!

Cut the tomatoes in chunks. Mix the vinegar, garlic, salt,
pepper, and basil; pour over tomatoes. Mix in the crumbled
Feta cheese. Refrigerate and marinate at least 4 hours
before serving.

*Preparation Time: 10 minutes*
*Marinating Time: 4 hours*

When making cream sauces, use evaporated skim milk instead
of heavy cream or half & half.

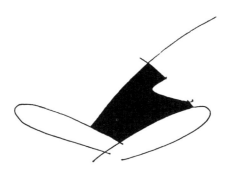

# Low-Fat Diet Plan for Day 9

*Breakfast:*
1 Lender's Bagel
1 tablespoon Polander All Fruit - any flavor
1 cup skim milk
1 small banana

*Lunch:*
2 ounces grilled chicken
Caesar Salad *
Croutons*
1 ounce whole wheat roll

*Snack:*
1 (8-ounce) Dannon sugar-free, nonfat vanilla yogurt
   (or your favorite flavor)

*Dinner:*
Pizza with Whole Wheat Crust* and
Sun-dried Tomato Sauce*
Greek Salad*

*Snack:*
Large apple

## CAESAR SALAD

*Free exchange—use without limiting quantity.*

1 package dry Caesar salad dressing mix
1/4 cup red wine vinegar (or your favorite vinegar)
1 tablespoon olive oil
1/2 cup water
2 tablespoons Light & Lively cottage cheese, creamed in
   blender
1 clove garlic

Mix all ingredients together and use freely on Romaine
or any other type of lettuce.

*Preparation Time: 5 minutes*

# CAESAR SALAD CROUTONS

*1 serving or 1/2 cup = 1 Bread Exchange.*
*70 calories per serving.*

French bread (stale bread is fine)
Pam cooking spray
Minced garlic, dry (to taste)
Hidden Valley Ranch dry salad dressing mix
Lemon pepper, to taste

Cut French bread in half lengthwise and spray with Pam. Sprinkle liberally with garlic, ranch dressing, and lemon pepper. Cube bread and place on nonstick baking sheet. Bake at 225° for 30 minutes or until dry.

*Preparation Time: 10 minutes*
*Cooking Time: 30 minutes*


# WHOLE WHEAT PIZZA DOUGH

*Makes 8 servings.*
*1 serving = 2 Bread Exchanges.*
*140 calories per serving.*

1 package of active dry yeast
1 teaspoon sugar
1 1/2 cups warm water, divided
1 1/2 cups all-purpose flour
1 1/2 cups whole wheat flour
2 teaspoons salt
1 teaspoon pepper
1 tablespoon olive oil
Pam cooking spray

In a small bowl, dissolve the yeast, sugar, and 1/2 cup of warm water. Let stand for 10 minutes. (The yeast mixture will become bubbly.) Set aside.

In a large mixing bowl, combine both flours, along with the salt and pepper. Add the dissolved yeast, oil, and remaining 1/2 cup of water.

Remove the dough and knead 8 to 10 minutes on a well floured board. Knead until smooth and pliable. Roll into a ball, and place the dough into a large bowl that has been sprayed well with Pam. Spray the dough with Pam and cover with plastic wrap. Place in a warm place

*continued*

for approximately 2 hours or until doubled in volume.

When dough has doubled, punch down and knead another 15 seconds. Using a rolling pin which has been floured, roll out dough on a well floured board. Transfer onto a pizza pan, sprinkled with cornmeal, add the Sun-Dried Tomato Sauce, any vegetables that you would like, and 2 cups of nonfat, part-skim Mozzarella cheese. Bake at 450° for 20 minutes.

*Preparation Time: 2 hours 30 minutes (to allow dough to rise)*
*Cooking Time: 20 minutes*


## SUN-DRIED TOMATO SAUCE

*Makes 5 servings.*
*1 serving = 2 Vegetable Exchanges.*
*40 calories per serving.*

1 1/4 cups water
1 package sun-dried tomatoes
2 (28-ounce) cans whole peeled tomatoes, undrained
3 cloves garlic, minced
1/2 yellow onion, chopped
3 ribs celery, minced
3 carrots, minced
Salt and pepper, to taste

Bring water to a boil. Add the sun-dried tomatoes and boil for 1 minute. Set aside—DO NOT discard the water.

In a nonstick saucepan that has been sprayed with Pam, pour the juice from the canned tomatoes, and sauté the garlic and onion in it for about 5 minutes. Add the sundried tomatoes with the water, the celery, and the carrots. Cook for 5 more minutes.

Chop the whole tomatoes with a food processor until chunky in texture. Add these, plus the salt and pepper to the saucepan. Simmer for 1 hour over low heat, stirring occasionally.

*Preparation Time: 25 minutes*
*Cooking Time: 1 hour*

# GREEK SALAD

*Makes 4 servings.*
*1 serving = 1 Fat, 1 Vegetable, and 1/2 Protein Exchange.*
*100 calories per serving.*

1 head iceberg lettuce, chopped well
1/2 cup red wine vinegar
1 tablespoon garlic powder
2 tablespoon oregano
1 teaspoon salt
1 teaspoon pepper
4 ounces Feta cheese

Wash and drain the lettuce and chop into bite-size pieces. Set aside. Combine the vinegar with the spices and pour over the lettuce. Crumble the Feta cheese on top, and mix well. May be served immediately, but is best if left standing for 1/2 hour beforehand.

*Preparation Time: 10 minutes*

---

# Low-Fat Diet Plan for Day 10

*Breakfast:*
1 ounce cereal
1 cup skim milk
2 tablespoons raisins

*Lunch:*
8 ounces yogurt of choice (nonfat, sugar-free)
1 cup berries
12 saltine crackers

*Snack:*
Small apple

*Dinner:*
Mexican Chicken*
1 1/2 cups rice
Marinated Cucumber Salad*

# MEXICAN CHICKEN

*Makes 4 servings.*
*1 serving = 4 Protein and 1 1/2 Vegetable Exchanges.*
*320 calories per serving.*

1 green pepper
1 onion
2 cloves garlic, minced
2 1/2 cups tomato sauce
3 tablespoons chili powder
1 tablespoon + 1 teaspoon cocoa
2 tablespoons + 2 teaspoons water
1 teaspoon parsley
4 (4-ounce) boneless, skinless chicken breasts

In a large nonstick skillet, sauté the green pepper, onion, and garlic. Add the tomato sauce and chili powder. Dissolve the cocoa in the water, and add to the tomato mixture. Add the chicken and simmer for 40 minutes with the lid on. Sprinkle with parsley.

*Preparation Time: 15 minutes*
*Cooking Time: 40 minutes*


# MARINATED CUCUMBER SALAD

*Free vegetable.*
*Use without limit.*

2 cucumbers, sliced
1 tomato, chopped
1/2 onion, coarsely chopped
2/3 cup seasoned rice vinegar
2 cloves garlic, pressed
1 teaspoon seasoned pepper
1/4 cup Feta cheese (optional)

Cut up cucumbers, tomato, and onion. Mix the vinegar, garlic, and pepper, and pour over the vegetables. Best if marinated overnight.

**Note:** If Feta cheese is used in the recipe, add 4 Protein Exchanges.

*Preparation Time: 10 minutes*

# Low-Fat Diet Plan for Day 11

*Breakfast :*
1 cup Squash with Cinnamon*
1 large apple, cut into slices and dipped into squash

*Lunch:*
1 cup brown rice
Sautéed vegetables
Marinated Mushrooms*

*Snack:*
Small banana

*Dinner:*
4 Stuffed Cabbage Rolls with Sauerkraut*
1 cup milk

## SQUASH WITH CINNAMON
*Makes 3 servings.*
*1 serving or 1/2 cup = 1 Bread Exchange.*
*70 calories per serving.*

1 (10-ounce) package acorn squash
1 teaspoon cinnamon
1 teaspoon pumpkin pie spice
1 teaspoon vanilla
2 packets Sweet & Low

Defrost squash, reserving liquid. In a saucepan, combine squash, cinnamon, spice, vanilla, and Sweet & Low. Bring to a boil, stirring constantly. Serve immediately.

*Preparation Time: 5 minutes*

If you want to cut out the sugar, use Sweet & Low instead of Equal. Equal is a protein and will denature in high heat. You will lose the sweetness once it is exposed to heat for a long duration.

# MARINATED MUSHROOMS
*Unlimited vegetable.*

**1 package fresh mushrooms**
**1/2 cup low-calorie Italian salad dressing**
**Freshly ground pepper (optional)**

Clean the mushrooms well and slice into halves. Pour the dressing over the mushrooms and refrigerate in a sealed container for at least 8 hours. The longer the mushrooms remain in the marinade, the better they will taste.

*Preparation Time: 15 minutes*
*Marinate Time: 8 hours or more*


# STUFFED CABBAGE ROLLS
# WITH SAUERKRAUT
*Makes 16 servings.*
*1 serving or 1 cabbage roll plus sauerkraut = 1 Protein,*
*    1/2 Bread, and 1 Vegetable Exchange.*
*130 calories per serving.*

**1 pound ground chuck (extra-lean)**
**4 cups white rice (cooked)**
**1 tablespoon garlic, crushed**
**2 large yellow onions, chopped**
**3 large (16-ounce) cans whole peeled tomatoes**
**1 teaspoon oregano**
**Salt and pepper, to taste**
**1 pound sauerkraut (use more if you like extra sauerkraut)**
**1 large head of cabbage**

In a nonstick skillet, cook the lean beef well done, draining off any excess grease as it cooks. Drain in a colander which has been lined with paper towels, and squeeze out any remaining grease. Set aside.

Cook the white rice according to the package directions. Set aside. Brown the garlic and onion in the tomato juice from the canned tomatoes, and combine it with the beef and rice. Add the oregano and salt and pepper. This is the stuffing for your cabbage rolls.

Crush the whole tomatoes in a food processor, and

*continued*

combine them with the sauerkraut. Set aside. Core the head of the cabbage and place it, core side down, into a pot of boiling water. As the cabbage cooks, peel off the leaves and set them aside. Continue until all of the leaves have been removed.

Place some of the sauerkraut mixture in a large casserole dish sprayed with Pam. Scoop a large amount of the rice/beef mixture and place it in 1 of the cabbage leaves. Fold the sides over and place the cabbage roll, seam side down, on top of the sauerkraut. Continue making cabbage rolls until all of the rice/beef mixture is gone. Any extra cabbage leaves can be shredded and placed on top of the layer of cabbage rolls. Place the remaining sauerkraut mixture over the cabbage rolls. Cook at 325° for 3 hours.

**Note:** These take a little extra effort to make, but are worth it! I use extra sauerkraut since it is a free food. You can make a pig of yourself with these and not have to worry about the calories. Also, these freeze very well.

*Preparation Time: 45 minutes*
*Cooking Time: 3 hours.*

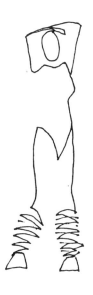

# Low-Fat Diet Plan for Day 12

*Breakfast:*
2 ounces cereal
1 cup skim milk
1/2 small banana
2 tablespoons raisins

*Lunch:*
Fajita with 1 ounce low-fat Cheddar cheese
Shredded lettuce, carrots, green peppers (and any
   other vegetable you want)
Salsa

*Snack:*
1 large apple

*Dinner:*
Chicken with Bouillon*
1 cup wild rice
Oven-Fried Zucchini Spears*

## CHICKEN WITH BOUILLON
*Makes 4 servings.*
*1 serving or 1 chicken breast = 4 Protein Exchanges.*
*280 calories per serving.*

4 (4-ounce) boneless, skinless chicken breasts
Italian seasonings
Lemon pepper
Garlic powder
Salt and pepper to taste
Basil (dry)
2 chicken bouillon cubes

Sprinkle chicken generously with spices on both sides.
In a nonstick pan sprayed with Pam, brown the chicken
on both sides on medium/high heat. Turn constantly to
prevent sticking. While the chicken is browning, dissolve the bouillon in one cup boiling water. When the
chicken is well-browned, add bouillon and lower tem-
perature to medium. Cover and cook another 30 minutes.

*Preparation Time: 5 minutes*
*Cooking Time: 40 minutes*

# FRIED ZUCCHINI SPEARS

*Makes 4 servings.*
*1 serving or 3 spears = 1 1/2 Vegetable, 1 Bread, 1 1/4*
*   Protein, and 1 Fat Exchange.*
*240 calories per serving.*

3 medium zucchini
1/3 cup corn meal
1/3 cup flour
1/4 cup Parmesan cheese
1/2 teaspoon onion powder
1/2 teaspoon garlic powder
1/8 teaspoon lemon pepper
1 egg, beaten
2 tablespoons milk

Preheat oven to 450°. Slice zucchini in half lenghtwise, and then half again. Roll the zucchini in a mixture of the egg and milk, and then dip it into a mixture of the flour and cornmeal, coating each spear thoroughly. Place on a cookie sheet sprayed with Pam, then spray each spear lightly with butter-flavored Pam. Bake 15 minutes or until zucchini is tender.

*Preparation Time: 15 minutes*
*Cooking Time: 15 minutes*

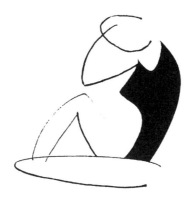

# Low-Fat Diet Plan for Day 13

*Breakfast:*
1/2 cup Fiber One Cereal (General Mills)
1 cup skim milk
1 cup fresh berries

*Lunch:*
2 servings Cabbage Salad with Noodles*
1 (2-ounce) whole wheat roll

*Snack:*
1 small banana

*Dinner:*
1 serving "Fried" Chicken*
1 serving Spiced Potatoes*
1 serving Spinach & Artichoke Casserole*

*Snack:*
1 cup cappuccino-flavored Dannon Yogurt (nonfat,
    sugar-free)


## CABBAGE SALAD WITH NOODLES
*Makes 12 servings.*
*1 serving = 1 Vegetable, 1/2 Fat and 1/3 Bread Exchange.*
*70 calories per serving.*

1 small head of cabbage, chopped into slivers
2 tablespoons sesame seeds, toasted
1 package low-fat chicken-flavored Ramen noodles, crushed

DRESSING:
Seasoning packet from Ramen noodles
1 teaspoon sesame oil
4 packets Sweet & Low
1/4 cup apple cider vinegar

Chop the cabbage into slivers and mix with the toasted
sesame seeds, along with the crushed noodles. Combine
the dressing ingredients and toss thoroughly through the
cabbage mixture. Serve immediately!

   **Note:** If kept overnight, the noodles will become soggy.
*Preparation Time: 20 minutes*

# FRIED CHICKEN

*Makes 6 servings.*
*1 serving or 1 breast = 4 1/2 Protein, 1/2 Bread, and 1/4*
   *Fat Exchange.*
*360 calories per serving.*

1/2 cup cornmeal
1/4 cup all-purpose flour
2 tablespoons grated Parmesan cheese
1 1/2 teaspoons Italian seasonings
1/4 teaspoon garlic salt
1/4 teaspoon pepper
6 (4-ounce) chicken breasts, boneless and skinless
1/3 cup skim milk

Heat oven to 375°. Combine cornmeal, flour, Parmesan cheese and seasonings. Dip the chicken into the milk, and then coat with the cornmeal mixture. Place on a nonstick cookie sheet and bake for 40 minutes or until crispy and golden brown.

*Preparation Time: 15 minutes*
*Cooking Time: 45 minutes*


# SPICED POTATOES

*Makes 6 servings.*
*1 serving = 1 Bread Exchange.*
*70 calories per serving.*

3 large baking potatoes, scrubbed and sliced into 1/8-inch
   medallions
Salt
Pepper
Lemon pepper
Basil
Rosemary
Cayenne (optional)

Preheat oven to 400°. Place potato slices on a nonstick baking sheet. Spray potato slices lightly with Pam, and then sprinkle with the spices. (Remember, the potato slices are very thin, so use spices sparingly.) Bake for 15 minutes or until tender and brown.

*Preparation Time: 10 minutes*
*Cooking Time: 15 minutes*

# SPINACH & ARTICHOKE CASSEROLE

*Makes 10 servings.*
*1 serving = 1 Vegetable and 1/4 Protein Exchange.*
*45 calories per serving—this is a very low-calorie entrée,*
  *so pig out to your heart's content!*

2 (10-ounce) packages frozen, chopped spinach, thawed
   and drained
2 (14-ounce) cans artichoke hearts, drained and chopped
1/2 cup chopped onion
1/2 cup low-fat cottage cheese, creamed (in blender)
1/2 teaspoon salt
3/4 teaspoon white pepper
Dash of cayenne
2 tablespoons Parmesan cheese

Chop spinach in a food processor. Set aside. Chop the
artichokes and add to spinach. Sauté onion in a large,
nonstick skillet with a little water until it becomes tender. Add the spinach and artichokes; mix well. Add the
remaining ingredients and place the mixture into a casserole dish sprayed with Pam. Heat at 350°, until casserole is heated through, approximately 10 minutes.

   **Note:** This recipe can be made a day or two ahead. If
you add 1 cup of cottage cheese (creamed), this dish can
be used as a dip.

*Preparation Time: 20 minutes*
*Cooking Time: 10 minutes*

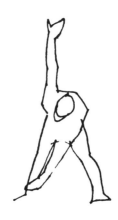

# Low-Fat Diet Plan for Day 14

*Breakfast:*
1 ounce cereal
1 cup skim milk
1 small banana

*Lunch:*
1 serving Sloppy Joes*
1 (2-ounce) hoagie roll
1 ounce low-fat cheese

*Dinner:*
1 serving Linguine with Puttanesca*
Salad with low-calorie dressing

*Snack:*
Large apple

## SLOPPY JOES
*Makes 8 servings.*
*1 serving = 2 Protein, 1/2 Vegetable and 1/4 Fat Ex-*
    *change.*
*175 calories per serving.*

**1 pound lean ground turkey**
**2 packages sloppy joe seasoning**
**2 (6-ounce) cans tomato paste**
**2 1/2 cups water**

Brown the turkey and drain well. Blot out any excess grease with a paper towel. Stir in the seasonings and tomato paste. Add the water and bring to a boil and simmer 15 minutes.

*Preparation Time: 5 minutes*
*Cooking Time: 20 minutes*

When baking, substitute applesauce or puréed fruit (i.e., pears) for the vegetable oil.

# LINGUINE WITH PUTTANESCA

*Makes 8 servings.*
*1 serving or 1 1/2 cups = 3 Bread, 1 Vegetable, and 1 Fat*
  *Exchange.*
*275 calories per serving.*

2 (28-ounce) cans whole peeled tomatoes, reserve liquid
1 large yellow onion, chopped
10 cloves garlic, minced
2 tablespoons tomato paste
1 tube anchovy paste
3/4 cup black olives, chopped
4 tablespoons capers, drained
2 teaspoons basil, dried
2 teaspoons oregano, dried
Dash of crushed red pepper flakes
Freshly ground black pepper
1 pound linguine

In a large saucepan sprayed with Pam, drain the juice
from the 2 cans of whole peeled tomatoes. Add the onion and garlic and cook over low heat for 10-15 minutes,
until tender. Crush the tomatoes into a chunky consis-
tency, and add them to the saucepan. Stir in the tomato
paste. Cook for 5 minutes over medium heat. Add the
anchovy paste, olives, capers, basil, oregano, red-pepper
flakes and black pepper. Mix well, and let simmer over
medium heat for 30 minutes. Stir occasionally.

Cook the linguine according to the package directions.
When the pasta is al dente, drain in a colander and toss
together with the Puttanesca sauce.

*Preparation Time: 20 minutes*
*Cooking Time: 45 minutes*

When making soup or gravy, skim off the fat, or put the broth
in the refrigerator so that the fat congeals and can be peeled
off. Also, a fat-skimming pitcher is available.

# Low-Fat Diet Plan for Day 15

**Breakfast:**
1/2 cup Fiber One Cereal
2 tablespoons raisins
1 cup skim milk

**Lunch:**
Pita Pocket filled with Grilled Vegetables*
1 cup skim milk
1 large apple

**Dinner:**
1 serving Lime & Honey Chicken*
Large Caesar Salad with Low-fat Caesar Salad Dressing* (See Index.)
1/2 cup Croutons (See Index.)
1 cup Spinach Pesto with Vermicelli* (Save some for lunch the next day.)

**Snack:**
1 small apple

## PITA POCKET
## FILLED WITH GRILLED VEGETABLES
*1 serving = 2 Bread and 4 Vegetable Exchanges.*
*230 calories per serving.*

1 small yellow onion
1 small green pepper
1 small red pepper
5 mushrooms, cleaned and sliced
Salt & pepper, to taste
1 whole wheat pita bread round
3 slices sweet pickle
1/2 tomato, sliced
1/2 cup shredded lettuce

Slice onion and peppers into strips. Clean and slice the mushrooms. Set aside. In a large, nonstick skillet sprayed with Pam, sauté onion, peppers, and mushrooms. Add salt and pepper to taste. If the vegetables start to stick, add a little water to the pan. Cook the vegetables until tender. Cut the pita bread in half, and stuff it with the cooked vegetables, sweet pickle, tomato, and lettuce.

# LIME & HONEY CHICKEN

*Makes 4 servings.*
*1 serving or 1 breast = 4 Protein and 1/2 Bread Exchange.*
*315 calories per serving.*

2 1/2 tablespoons honey
2 tablespoons lime juice
1 1/2 tablespoons grainy mustard
1/4 teaspoon lemon pepper
1/4 teaspoon freshly ground black pepper
Salt (to taste)
4 (4-ounce) chicken breasts, boneless and skinless

Mix together the honey, lime, mustard, and spices. Pour over the chicken and marinate at least 3 hours. Remove the chicken from the marinade, reserving the juice, and brown the chicken on high heat in a nonstick skillet sprayed with Pam, for approximately 8 minutes. Turn the chicken every few minutes so that both sides brown evenly. Season with extra lemon pepper if desired. Pour remaining marinade over the chicken and reduce the heat, cover, and simmer for 30 minutes.

*Preparation Time: 10 minutes*
*Marinate Time: 3 hours*
*Cooking Time: 40 minutes*


# SPINACH PESTO WITH VERMICELLI

*Makes 6 servings.*
*1 serving = 1 Vegetable, 2 Breads, 1/4 Fat Exchange.*
*200 calories per serving.*

1 (10-ounce) box chopped frozen spinach, thawed and
    drained
1 tablespoon basil
15 ounces marinara sauce (Di Giorgno Low-fat Sauce)
12 ounces vermicelli

Cream spinach in food processor. Mix together with basil and sauce. Cook pasta according to package directions, drain and toss with sauce.

**Note:** Remove spinach from freezer the night before, and place it in a bowl to ensure none of the liquid is lost.

*Preparation Time: 15 minutes*
*Cooking Time: 15 minutes*

# Low-Fat Diet Plan for Day 16

**Breakfast:**
1 ounce cereal
1 cup skim milk
1 large banana

**Lunch:**
Pita Pizza*
1 8-ounce Dannon sugar-free, nonfat yogurt
1 large apple

**Dinner:**
4 ounce chicken breast with Barbecue Sauce*
Cole Slaw*
Large baked potato


## PITA PIZZA

*1 serving or whole pizza = 2 Bread, 2 Protein, and 1
    Vegetable Exchange.*
*205 calories per serving.*

1 pita bread, split into two rounds
Pesto sauce, optional (reserved from the night before)
1 large tomato, sliced thin
1 teaspoon Italian spices
1/2 teaspoon garlic powder
Salt and pepper, to taste
1 ounce low-fat cheese, grated

Slice the pita bread in half horizontally, making two cir-
cular halves. Toast very slightly in toaster oven. Place
the pesto sauce, tomato and seasoning on the halves. Top
the rounds with grated cheese and return to toaster oven.
Toast until the cheese is melted.

**Note:** Any kind of vegetable may be put on the pizza.
For example, defrosted broccoli and spinach or chopped
green and red peppers.

Instead of frying in a pan with oil or butter, "fry" foods in the
oven at very high heat.

# BARBECUE SAUCE

*Makes 10 servings or 1 quart.*
*1 serving or 1/4 cup = 1 Bread Exchange.*
*70 calories per serving.*

12 cloves garlic, crushed
2 medium onions, chopped
2 cups Heinz ketchup
1/4 cup brown sugar or equivalent Sweet & Low brown
    sugar
4 teaspoons basil
1/2 cup lemon juice
1/2 teaspoon tabasco
1 teaspoon pepper
1/2 cup chili powder

In a large saucepan, cook the garlic and onions with 1/4 cup water until it clarifies. Add all of the remaining ingredients, and bring the sauce to a boil. Simmer for 5 minutes.

*Preparation Time: 10 minutes*
*Cooking Time: 15 minutes*


# COLE SLAW

*Makes 6 servings.*
*1 serving or 1 cup = 1 Vegetable and 1 Fat Exchange.*
*60 calories per serving.*

1 head cabbage, shredded
1 teaspoon cinnamon
1/4 cup + 2 tablespoons Miracle Whip Light
1/4 cup + 2 tablespoons red wine vinegar
1/2 teaspoon salt
1/2 teaspoon pepper
6 packets Sweet & Low

Shred the cabbage and put into a large mixing bowl. Combine the remaining ingredients and mix in with the cabbage. Let stand at least 4 hours.

*Preparation Time: 15 minutes*
*Marinate Time: 4 hours or more*

# Low-Fat Diet Plan for Day 17

*Breakfast:*
1 ounce oatmeal
1 small apple
2 tablespoons raisins
1/2 cup skim milk

*Lunch:*
1 (6-inch diameter) pita bread stuffed with Marinated Cucumber Salad (See Index.)
1 cup skim milk

*Dinner:*
1 serving Orange Chicken with Broccoli*
Marinated Mushrooms (Unlimited. See Index.)
1 serving Lemon & Lime Jello Mold*
1 1/2 cups rice

## ORANGE CHICKEN WITH BROCCOLI

*Makes 6 servings.*
*1 serving or 1 breast = 4 Protein and 1 Vegetable Exchange.*
*305 calories per serving.*

6 (4-ounce) chicken breasts, boned and skinned
1 1/2 cups sugar-free orange flavored soda (carbonated)
1/2 cup soy sauce
2 packages frozen chopped broccoli spears, thawed

Marinate the chicken in the orange soda and soy sauce for at least 8 hours. Place the chicken and marinade in a baking dish and cover. Cook at 350° for 1 hour. Baste the chicken occasionally. After the chicken has been cooking for 45 minutes, add the thawed broccoli and finish cooking the two together for the remaining 15 minutes. Serve over rice.

*Preparation Time: 5 minutes*
*Marinate Time: 8 hours*
*Cooking Time: 1 hour*

# LEMON & LIME JELLO MOLD

*Makes 5 servings.*
*1 serving = 1/2 Milk and 1 Fruit Exchange.*
*105 calories per serving.*

1 small package (0.3 ounce) Lime Sugar-Free Jello
1 small package (0.3 ounce) Lemon Sugar-Free Jello
1 cup boiling water
1 (20-ounce) can crushed unsweetened pineapple (with the
    juice)
3 cups Dannon Light Vanilla Yogurt (nonfat, sugar-free)

Combine the lemon and lime jello with the 1 cup of boiling water until dissolved well. Add the can of crushed
pineapple with the juice and mix in the yogurt. Stir
until all ingredients are mixed well. Refrigerate for 1
1/2 hours before serving.

**Note:** You can make many variations of this recipe,
using different types of fruit and jello. For instance, try
2 packages of strawberry-banana jello and a frozen package of strawberries, thawed, reserving the juice.

*Preparation Time: 10 minutes*
*Marinate Time: 1 1/2 hours*

It is much better to show restraint in the grocery store than it
is once you have the "irresistible" food in your house.

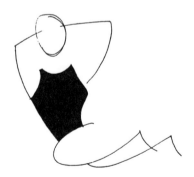

# Low-Fat Diet Plan for Day 18

*Breakfast:*
1 (8-ounce) carton yogurt (nonfat, sugar-free)
3/4 cup strawberries
1/2 cup blueberries

*Lunch:*
1 English Muffin Pizza*
1 cup skim milk
1 small salad with low-calorie dressing

*Snack:*
1 small banana

*Dinner:*
Sweet & Sour Chicken*
1 cup rice
Pea Salad* (Note: Save some for next day's lunch.)

*Snack:*
1 Fudgsicle (Good Humor Brand—sugar-free, nonfat)


## ENGLISH MUFFIN PIZZA
*Makes 1 serving.*
*1 serving = 2 Bread and 1 Protein Exchange.*
*210 calories per serving.*

**1 whole wheat English muffin**
**1 small tomato, sliced thin**
**Italian spices**
**Salt and pepper, to taste**
**1 ounce low-fat, part-skim Mozzarella cheese, shredded**

Split the English muffin in half and lightly toast. Place thin slices of tomato on each, and sprinkle with Italian spices. Add salt and pepper to taste. Top with shredded cheese. Toast again until the cheese is melted.

*Preparation Time: 5 minutes*

# SWEET & SOUR CHICKEN

*Makes 4 servings.*
*1 serving or 1 breast = 4 Protein and 1/2 Bread Exchange.*
*315 calories per serving.*

1 onion, thinly sliced
2 cloves garlic, minced
4 (4-ounce) chicken breasts, skinned and boned
1/2 cup red wine vinegar
1 teaspoon + 1 tablespoon soy sauce
3 tablespoons honey
2 teaspoons yellow mustard
1/2 cup tomato juice

Thinly slice and sauté onion and garlic in a nonstick pan sprayed with Pam. If it starts to stick, add 1 tablespoon water. Set aside.

In a separate nonstick pan, braise the chicken in vinegar, soy, honey, mustard and tomato juice. Top with the browned onion and cook 40 minutes with the lid on.

*Preparation Time: 20 minutes*
*Cooking Time: 40 minutes*


# PEA SALAD

*Makes 4 servings.*
*1 serving = 3/4 Bread, 3/4 Vegetable and 1 Fat exchange.*
*125 calories per serving.*

1 head lettuce, finely chopped
1 (10-ounce) package frozen peas, thawed
1/2 red onion, chopped
4 tablespoons Miracle Whip Light
3 tablespoons water

Mix the lettuce, peas, and onion. Combine the Miracle Whip and water, and pour over the lettuce mixture. Toss well and let stand 4 hours or more.

**Note:** May be eaten immediately, but is best if let to stand a few hours.

*Preparation Time: 5 minutes*
*Marinate Time: 4 hours or more*

# Low-Fat Diet Plan for Day 19

*Breakfast:*
1 (8-ounce) nonfat, sugar-free carton yogurt
1 large apple, sliced into sections to dip in yogurt

*Snack:*
Small banana

*Lunch:*
Pita bread with Pea Salad* (Left over from evening
   before, or see Index.)
1 cup skim milk

*Dinner:*
1 serving Turkey Sausage & Peppers* with pasta
Large mixed green salad with Italian Salad Dressing*

## TURKEY SAUSAGE & PEPPERS
*Makes 4 servings.*
*1 serving = 4 Protein, 3 1/2 Bread, and 2 Vegetable
   Exchanges.*
*565 calories per serving.*

16 ounces ground turkey, extra-lean
2/3 cup Italian bread crumbs
2 teaspoons onion powder
1 1/4 teaspoons fennel seeds, crushed
3/4 teaspoon garlic powder, divided
1/4 teaspoon salt (optional)
1 1/4 teaspoons crushed red pepper
2 1/2 tablespoons water
2 1/2 cups sweet red and green bell pepper strips
1 (16-ounce) can whole tomatoes, broken up
1 1/2 teaspoons oregano leaves, crushed
12 ounces penne or other tubular pasta, cooked

In a large bowl, combine turkey, bread crumbs, onion
powder, fennel seeds, 1/4 teaspoon garlic powder, salt,
red pepper and water. With your hands, form the mixture into 1-inch meatballs.

   Spray a large nonstick skillet with Pam. Add the meatballs and cook them, turning occasionally until well-

*continued*

browned and cooked through. This should take approximately 8-10 minutes. Remove skillet from heat and carefully remove meatballs, using a slotted spoon.

Spray skillet again with cooking spray, and add sweet peppers. Cook and stir until crisp-tender—approximately 5 minutes. Stir in tomatoes, oregano and remaining 1/4 teaspoon garlic powder. Return meatballs to the skillet. Bring to a boil, reduce heat and simmer, uncovered, until sauce has thickened and meatballs are heated through—about 5 minutes. Add approximately 1/2 teaspoon sugar to the sauce, if needed. Serve with pasta.

*Preparation Time: 30 minutes*
*Cooking Time: 40 minutes*

## ITALIAN SALAD DRESSING
*Free food.*
*Use is unlimited.*

2/3 cup rice vinegar (Marukan, seasoned gourmet)
2 cloves garlic, pressed
1 teaspoon seasoned black pepper
1 teaspoon Italian spices

Combine all ingredients and serve immediately.

# Low-Fat Diet Plan for Day 20

*Breakfast:*
1 ounce cereal
1 small banana
1 cup skim milk

*Lunch:*
Potato Pancake Pizza*
1 cup skim milk

*Snack:*
1 small apple

*Dinner:*
Sweet & Sour Pork*
Applesauce*

# POTATO PANCAKE PIZZAS

*Makes 4 servings.*
*1 serving or 1 cup = 1 Bread and 1/4 Protein Exchange.*
*90 calories per serving.*

3 medium potatoes
2 garlic cloves, minced
1/4 cup grated onion
3 egg whites, well-beaten
1/2 teaspoon salt (optional)
1/4 teaspoon pepper
1 large tomato, thinly sliced
4 ounces low-fat, part-skim Mozzarella cheese

In a food processor, chop the potatoes, place on a paper towel, and sprinkle lightly with salt to draw the water out. Let stand 10 minutes, blotting off any excess fluid.

Sauté garlic and onion in nonstick pan approximately 5 minutes or until tender and brown. If the onion starts to stick, add a little water to the pan. Combine onion, potato, egg whites, salt and pepper. Mix well.

Prepare pancakes by placing 1/2 cup portions into a nonstick skillet and cook until golden brown—approximately 15 to 20 minutes.

To make a potato pizza, add a slice of tomato on top of the potato pancake, and cover with 1/2 ounce of cheese. Cover the skillet to allow the cheese to melt.

*Preparation Time: 20 minutes*
*Cooking Time: 15 to 20 minutes*

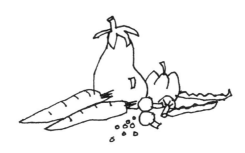

# SWEET & SOUR PORK

*Makes 3 servings.*
*1 serving = 4 Protein, 1 Fruit, and 1/2 Vegetable Exchange.*
*230 calories per serving.*

12 ounces extra-lean boneless pork, cubed
1 tablespoon taco seasoning
1/3 cup Polander Peach Preserves
8 ounces chunky salsa (mild/medium)
1 1/2 teaspoons parsley

Brown the pork in a nonstick skillet until fully cooked. Mix the remaining ingredients in a bowl and blend well. Pour the mixture over the pork and simmer for 10 minutes. Serve over rice.

*Preparation Time: 10 minutes*
*Cooking Time: 10 minutes*


# APPLESAUCE

*Makes 6 servings.*
*1 serving or 1/2 cup = 1 Fruit Exchange.*
*40 calories per serving.*

6 large apples
1 cup water
1 tablespoon cinnamon
4 packets Sweet & Low
1 tablespoon vanilla

Core and skin the apples. Cut into bite-size chunks. Place the apples and water in a large saucepan, and bring them to a boil, keeping the lid on. Add the cinnamon and Sweet & Low and let simmer on low heat, uncovered, for 30 minutes, stirring occasionally, until thickened. Remove from the heat and add the vanilla extract.

*Preparation Time: 20 minutes*
*Cooking Time: 30 minutes*

Just because it is fat-free doesn't mean there are no calories. Count those calories!

# Low-Fat Diet Plan for Day 21

*Breakfast:*
1 ounce cereal
2 tablespoons raisins
1 cup skim milk

*Snack:*
1 small banana

*Lunch:*
Vegetable Pita Pizzas*
Small salad
1 cup skim milk
1 small apple

*Dinner:*
Cabbage Casserole*
1 (2-ounce) whole wheat roll

*Snack:*
2 Fudgsicles (sugar-free, Good Humor Brand)


## VEGETABLE PITA PIZZAS

*Makes 1 serving.*
*1 serving = 2 Bread, 2 Vegetable, and 2 Protein Exchanges.*
*315 calories per serving.*

1 (6-inch) whole wheat pita
1 tomato, sliced
Italian spices
Salt and pepper to taste
Vegetables of your choice
1 ounce shredded low-fat Muenster cheese
1 ounce Feta cheese

Split the pita in half, making two rounds. Place the sliced tomato (or tomato sauce), Italian spices, salt and pepper, and any other vegetables (such as broccoli, mushrooms, or green peppers) on top. Put 1 ounce of low-fat cheese on each half. Place on a toaster oven tray, or under the broiler in the oven, and toast until the cheese is melted.

*Preparation Time: 5 minutes*
*Cooking Time: 5 minutes*

# CABBAGE CASSEROLE

*Makes 8 servings.*
*1 serving = 2 Protein and 4 Vegetable Exchanges.*
*215 calories per serving.*

2 heads cabbage, sliced
1 onion, chopped
1 pound ground turkey, extra-lean
1 (6-ounce) can tomato paste
1 teaspoon salt
1/2 tablespoon pepper
1/4 teaspoon cayenne (optional)

Cut the cabbage into 1/8-inch slices and chop the onion coarsely. Place the cabbage and onion in boiling water. While cabbage is cooking, brown and drain the turkey. When the cabbage and onion are wilted, drain them well and place them in a large pot. Add the turkey and the rest of the ingredients and mix well.

Simmer for 10 minutes at medium heat, stirring occasionally. Serve immediately.

*Preparation Time: 20 minutes*
*Cooking Time: 25 minutes*

# Low-Fat Diet Plan for Day 22

*Breakfast:*
1 serving Rice Pudding*

*Lunch:*
Egg Salad* with lettuce and tomato
2 slices whole wheat bread
1 cup skim milk

*Snack:*
1 small banana

*Dinner:*
2 servings Zucchini Casserole*
1 serving Potato Pancakes* (See Index.)

*Snack:*
1 small apple

# RICE PUDDING

*Makes 4 servings.*
*1 serving = 1 Bread, 3/4 Milk, 1/4 Protein Exchange.*
*140 calories per serving.*

2 cups cooked rice (Minute Rice)
1 (12-ounce) can evaporated skim milk
4 packets Sweet & Low
1 teaspoon vanilla
1 teaspoon cinnamon
1 egg + 2 egg whites (beaten)

Cook the instant rice according to the package directions, leaving out any butter it may suggest. Make enough to yield 2 cups. Refrigerate the rice for 1 hour or until rice is cold.

In a large, nonstick saucepan, combine the evaporated skim milk, Sweet & Low, vanilla, and cinnamon, stirring constantly until it comes to a boil. Beat the egg and egg whites. Add a little bit of the hot milk mixture to the egg—a tablespoonful at a time—to warm the egg slowly. After the beaten eggs have been heated, add the cold rice to the hot milk mixture, stirring constantly. When the rice is mixed in well, add the warmed egg. Cook over medium/high heat, stirring continuously, for approximately 5 minutes, or until thickened. If the rice starts to stick to the pan, lower the heat. Eat immediately while warm or refrigerate for later. The pudding will thicken more as it cools in the refrigerator.

**Note:** This is a great way to use leftover rice.

*Preparation Time: 5 minutes to prepare and 1 hour to refrigerate the rice before making the recipe.*
*Cooking Time: 10 minutes*

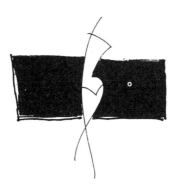

# EGG SALAD

*1 serving = 1 1/2 Protein Exchanges.*
*105 calories per serving.*

3 egg whites, chopped
1/2 cup cottage cheese
1 tablespoon mustard
1/2 teaspoon paprika
1/4 cup onion or scallions, chopped

Hard-boil three eggs. Remove the yolks and discard. Chop
the egg whites and combine with remaining ingredients.
Serve immediately on a sandwich or in a salad.

*Preparation Time: 10 minutes*


# ZUCCHINI CASSEROLE

*Makes 9 servings.*
*1 serving = 1 Bread, 1/2 Protein, 1/2 Fat, 1 1/2 Vegetable*
  *Exchanges.*
*165 calories per serving.*

3 chicken bouillon cubes
3 pounds zucchini
1 cup low-fat cottage cheese, creamed in the blender
3 cups mushrooms (8 ounces), chopped
1 can 99% fat-free cream of chicken soup
1 onion, grated
1 carrot, grated
3/4 cup skim milk
1 cup low-fat Cheddar cheese, grated
2 cups saltine crackers, crushed (14-ounce package)
1 teaspoon basil
1 teaspoon parsley
1/2 teaspoon garlic powder
1/2 teaspoon salt
1/2 teaspoon pepper
1 teaspoon Season All

Preheat oven to 350°. In a large pot, half-filled with water, add the 3 bouillon cubes and bring to a rolling boil.
Dice the zucchini and add to the boiling water until par-
boiled (about 7 minutes, or until a fork may be inserted).
Remove the zucchini, drain, and set aside.

*continued*

In a large bowl, combine the creamed cottage cheese, chopped mushrooms, fat-free chicken soup, grated onion, grated carrot, skim milk, and grated low-fat cheese. Set aside.

In a blender, or with a rolling pin, crush the package of saltines and season with the spices.

Mix together the zucchini, the cottage cheese mixture and the seasoned saltine crumbs. Pour into a large, Pam-sprayed casserole dish and cook at 350° for 30 minutes.

**Note:** Bread crumbs may be used, but will increase the overall number of calories.

*Preparation Time: 30 minutes*
*Cooking Time: 30 minutes*

# Low-Fat Diet Plan for Day 23

*Breakfast:*
Omelet with Tomato & Cheese*
2 slices whole wheat toast
1 tablespoon Polander All Fruit (any flavor)

*Lunch:*
1/2 (6-inch) pita pocket stuffed with grilled veg-
    etables and low-calorie dressing
1 (8-ounce) yogurt (nonfat and sugar-free—
    cappuccino flavor by Dannon is excellent!)
1 small banana

*Dinner:*
2 servings Feta & Spinach Quiche*
2 ounces French bread
Salad with low-calorie dressing

*Snack:*
1 small apple

To expend 100 calories, you have to walk or run 1 mile.

# OMELET WITH TOMATO & CHEESE

*1 serving = 2 1/2 Protein, 1/2 Fat, and 1 Vegetable Exchange.*
*220 calories per serving.*

1 whole egg + 2 egg whites
2 tablespoons skim milk
1 small tomato, chopped
1 tablespoon chives, chopped (optional)
Salt and pepper, to taste
1 ounce low-fat Swiss cheese (or your favorite variety)

Beat together the whole egg, egg whites, and 2 tablespoons skim milk. Heat a nonstick skillet, coat it lightly with Pam, and pour in the egg mixture. Lift the sides of the cooked egg away from the pan as the egg starts to set. Let any uncooked egg run over the edge onto the pan. As the egg is cooking, chop up a small tomato and a few chives (if desired), and place them on half of the omelet. Season with salt and pepper if desired. Place the cheese on the tomato and fold the other half of the omelet over. Cover the pan and remove from the heat for 1 minute. Serve immediately.

*Preparation Time: 5 minutes*
*Cooking Time: 5 minutes*


# FETA & SPINACH QUICHE

*Makes 5 servings.*
*1 serving = 1 Protein, 1/2 Milk, 1/2 Bread, 1 Vegetable, and 1/2 Fat Exchange.*
*185 calories per serving.*

1 (10-ounce) package frozen, chopped spinach (thawed and well drained)
2 cups skim milk
4 egg whites, beaten well
2 ounces Feta cheese
2 ounces low-fat Swiss cheese
1 package Knorr's Vegetable Soup Mix

Preheat oven to 375°. Defrost and drain the spinach well. In a large mixing bowl, combine the spinach, milk, egg whites, both cheeses, and the Knorr's Vegetable Soup Mix.

*continued*

Spray a 9-inch pie pan or quiche dish well with Pam cooking spray. Pour the quiche mixture into the dish and bake 40 minutes or until set and knife inserted in the center comes out clean.

*Preparation Time: 15 minutes*
*Cooking Time: 40 minutes*

# Low-Fat Diet Plan for Day 24

*Breakfast:*
Dannon vanilla sugar-free, nonfat yogurt with 1/2
    teaspoon cinnamon mixed in
1 large apple, cut into slices (for dipping)
1/2 English muffin with
1 tablespoon Polander Fruit Spread (any variety)

*Lunch:*
Melted Cheese Sandwich (toast 2 slices of whole
    wheat bread with 1 ounce low-fat cheese between
    them. Add lettuce, tomato, and mustard.)
Large dill pickle
1 cup skim milk

*Dinner:*
Sesame Chicken*
1 1/2 cups brown rice
Mixed green salad with low-calorie dressing

*Snack:*
Large orange

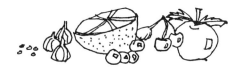

# SESAME CHICKEN

*Makes 4 servings.*
*1 serving or 1 breast = 4 Protein, 1/4 Bread, and 1/2 Fat
    Exchange.*
*325 calories per serving.*

1/2 cup soy sauce
1 teaspoon cinnamon
1 teaspoon ginger
1 teaspoon garlic powder
2 scallions, chopped
4 (4-ounce) chicken breasts, boneless and skinless
2 tablespoons flour
3 tablespoons sesame seeds
1/2 teaspoon salt
1/4 teaspoon pepper
1 teaspoon parsley

Combine the soy sauce, cinnamon, ginger, garlic powder,
and scallions. Marinate the chicken in this mixture for
at least 2 hours (preferably 8 hours).

Combine the flour, sesame seeds, salt, pepper, and parsley. Remove the chicken from the soy mixture, discard-
ing the marinade, and coat it thoroughly with the flour
mixture. Place on a nonstick cookie sheet sprayed with
Pam, and spray the chicken, too, lightly with the cooking
spray. Bake at 400° for 40 minutes.

*Preparation Time: 2 hours to marinate + 5 minutes to
    prepare coating mixture.*
*Cooking Time: 40 minutes.*

 Not all chicken is created equal. The dark meat has signifi-
cantly more calories and cholesterol than the white meat.

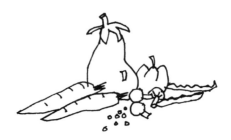

# Low-Fat Diet Plan for Day 25

*Breakfast:*
2 slices whole wheat toast
1 tablespoon Polander All Fruit
1 cup skim milk

*Lunch:*
Pita pizza (1 whole wheat pita split in half and
    toasted with thinly sliced tomato, Italian spices,
    salt and pepper, and 1 ounce shredded low-fat
    cheese melted on top.)
Small salad with low-calorie Italian dressing

*Snack:*
1 small banana

*Dinner:*
1 serving Veal & Peppers*
Mixed green salad with low-calorie dressing
1 cup skim milk


## VEAL & PEPPERS
*Makes 6 servings.*
*1 serving or 1 cutlet = 4 Protein, 1 Vegetable, and 1/2*
    *Bread Exchange.*
*340 calories per serving.*

2 tablespoons fresh garlic, minced
2 large onions, sliced
2 large green peppers, cut into strips
2 cups fresh mushrooms, cleaned and sliced
6 (4-ounce) veal cutlets
1 cup Catsup (Heinz)
1 cup water
1 tablespoon Worcestershire sauce
Salt and pepper, to taste

Preheat oven to 350°. In a nonstick skillet, sauté 1 tablespoon of garlic. Chop the onions, green peppers, and mushrooms, and add to the garlic. Sauté until tender. (Add a
little water to the pan if the vegetables start to stick.)
Set aside.

*continued*

In another sauté pan sprayed with Pam, brown the remaining garlic with 1 tablespoon water. Add the veal and cook until it is browned on both sides, turning occasionally. Set aside.

In a large casserole pan sprayed with Pam, line the vegetables in the bottom. Place the veal cutlets over the vegetables. Combine the catsup, water, Worcestershire sauce, salt and pepper to taste, and pour over the veal and vegetables.

Cover the casserole and cook for 45 minutes at 350°.

**Note:** May use chicken if preferred.

*Preparation Time: 20 minutes.*
*Cooking Time: 45 minutes.*

# Low-Fat Diet Plan for Day 26

*Breakfast:*
1 ounce cereal
1 cup skim milk
1 small banana

*Lunch:*
12 saltine crackers
1 ounce low-fat Cheddar cheese
1 large apple, cut into slices

*Snack:*
3 cups air-popped popcorn (Spray with butter-flavored Pam and salt lightly, if desired.)

*Dinner:*
1 serving Southwestern Chicken*
1 cup rice
Large mixed green salad with low-calorie dressing
1 cup skim milk
Steamed broccoli seasoned with lemon pepper, garlic, salt and pepper

# SOUTHWESTERN CHICKEN

*Makes 4 servings.*
*1 serving or 1 breast = 4 Protein and 1/2 Bread Exchange.*
*315 calories per serving.*

6 tablespoons catsup
6 tablespoons soy sauce
2 tablespoons Italian seasonings
1 teaspoon black pepper
1 teaspoon garlic powder
4 (4-ounce) chicken breasts, skinless and boneless

Mix together the catsup, soy sauce and spices. Set aside. Place chicken breasts in a nonstick skillet sprayed with Pam and brown on medium/high heat, turning occasionally to insure even browning. Pour the marinade over the chicken, and decrease heat to medium. Continue to cook with the lid on for 30 minutes.

**Note:** This is an excellent marinade for all meat and poultry. Use this to marinate your meat before grilling. Also, it is delicious served warm as a salad dressing.

*Preparation Time: 5 minutes.*
*Cooking Time: 35 to 40 minutes.*

Whip 1% low-fat cottage cheese in a blender and use it instead of sour cream in dips. This can also be used in baking breads instead of the oil.

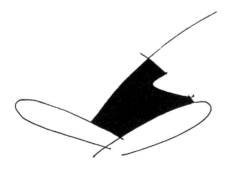

# Low-Fat Diet Plan for Day 27

*Breakfast:*
2 ounces cereal
1 cup skim milk

*Lunch:*
Vegetable sandwich (2 slices of your favorite whole
  grain bread with mustard, sliced tomatoes, shredded lettuce, shredded carrot, sliced cucumbers, and
  sliced mushrooms)
1 cup skim milk

*Snack:*
1 large apple

*Dinner:*
1 serving Chili* (Save some for the next day's lunch.)
1 (2-ounce) roll
Large green salad with low-calorie dressing

*Snack:*
1 large orange

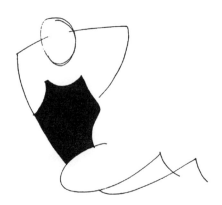

# CHILI

*Makes 8 servings.*
*1 serving or 1 cup = 4 Proteins, 1 Fat, and 1 Vegetable*
*   Exchange.*
*345 calories per serving.*

2 pounds extra-lean ground chuck, browned
2 large onions, chopped
1 large green pepper, chopped
4 cloves garlic, minced
4 tablespoons chili powder
1/2 teaspoon cayenne pepper
2 (6-ounce) cans tomato paste
1/2 cup white vinegar
1 (8-ounce) can tomato sauce
1/2 teaspoon oregano
1 (16-ounce) can whole tomatoes, chopped
1 teaspoon salt
1/4 teaspoon crushed red pepper flakes
1 1/2 teaspoons cumin
4 cups water

In a large skillet, brown the beef. Drain off any excess grease. Place the cooked beef on a paper towel, and blot out any remaining grease. Add the onions, green pepper, garlic; sauté with the meat. When the vegetables are tender, pour the entire meat/vegetable mixture in a very large pot.

Add the chili powder, cayenne pepper, tomato paste, vinegar, tomato sauce, oregano, whole tomatoes, salt, red pepper flakes, and water. Bring to a boil, then reduce to a simmer. Let mixture cook 1 1/2 hours, stirring occasionally. Before serving, skim off any excess fat and discard. Garnish with chopped onions, shredded cheese, and chopped lettuce.

*Preparation Time: 25 minutes*
*Cooking Time: 1 hour 30 minutes*

Saute with chicken broth, vegetable broth, white wine, or V-8 juice instead of butter or oil.

# Low-Fat Diet Plan for Day 28

*Breakfast:*
1 Popover*
1 cup skim milk
1 tablespoon raisins
1/2 small banana

*Lunch:*
Chili Salad (Shred 1/4 head lettuce and top with 1/2
    cup of Chili from day before.)
1 cup skim milk

*Snack:*
1 large orange

*Dinner:*
1 serving Chicken & Broccoli with Pasta*
Large green salad with low-calorie dressing

## POPOVERS
*Makes 6 servings.*
*1 serving or 1 giant popover = 1 1/2 Bread, 1/4 Milk,*
    *and 1/3 Protein Exchange.*
*150 calories per serving.*

1 1/2 cups all-purpose flour
1 1/2 cups skim milk
1 egg + 4 egg whites
1 teaspoon vanilla
1 teaspoon salt

Preheat oven to 425°. Place the popover pans in the oven
as it is warming up, allowing them to become very hot
before the batter is added.

In a large mixing bowl, combine all of the ingredients.
Mix together with a wire whisk until the batter is smooth.
Fill the preheated popover pans 3/4 full. Bake for 20
minutes at 425°, then reduce the heat to 350° for another
20 minutes.

*Preparation Time: 5 minutes*
*Cooking Time: 40 minutes*

# CHICKEN & BROCCOLI WITH PASTA

*Makes 4 servings.*
*1 serving = 4 Protein, 4 1/2 Bread, and 1 Vegetable*
  *Exchange.*
*615 calories per serving.*

12 ounces skinless and boneless chicken, cut into strips
1 medium green or red bell pepper
1 medium onion, chopped
1 1/2 cups broccoli flowerets
1 (10 3/4-ounce) can 99% fat-free cream of chicken soup
  (Campbell's, Healthy Request)
1 (10 3/4- ounce) can 99% fat-free cream of broccoli soup
  (Campbell's, Healthy Request.)
1/2 cup water
1 tablespoon basil
1/2 cup low-fat sharp Cheddar cheese
8 ounces noodles

In a nonstick skillet sprayed with Pam, brown the strips of chicken, turning them constantly, over medium/high heat. Set aside. In a separate skillet, cook the red pepper and onion until almost tender, and then add the broccoli. In a large casserole dish, combine the vegetables and chicken, and then add the soups, water, basil, and 1/2 of the cheese. Set aside.

Cook the pasta according to the package directions, drain, and then combine with the chicken mixture in the casserole. Top off with the remaining 1/4 cup of cheese and warm in a 375° oven for 15 minutes, until the cheese is melted.

*Preparation Time: 25 minutes*
*Cooking Time: 15 minutes*

Add chicken bouillon to the water instead of plain salt when making pasta and rice.

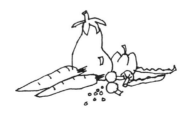

# Low-Fat Diet Plan for Day 29

*Breakfast:*
2 Low-Fat Southern Spoon Rolls*
2 tablespoons Polander All Fruit, any flavor

*Lunch:*
1 cup skim milk
1 Lender's Bagel with
2 servings Mushroom Pate*

*Snack:*
Small apple

*Dinner:*
1 serving Artichoke Chicken*
2 servings Spinach-Strawberry Salad*

*Snack:*
Nonfat, sugar-free yogurt


## LOW-FAT SOUTHERN SPOON ROLLS
*Makes 2 dozen rolls.*
*1 serving or 1 roll – 1 Bread Exchange.*
*80 calories per roll.*

3 packages double acting yeast
2 cups warm water
1 cup Light & Lively 1% Fat cottage cheese, creamed
1 cup unsweetened applesauce
10 packets Sweet & Low
3 egg whites
2 cups whole wheat flour
2 cups white flour
1 teaspoon salt
2 teaspoons baking powder

Dissolve the yeast in the warm water, and set aside. Place the cottage cheese in a blender and blend until smooth. Add the applesauce, Sweet & Low, and egg whites. Mix well and set aside. Combine the wheat flour, white flour, salt, and baking powder. Alternately add the flour mixture and the yeast mixture to the cottage cheese. Refrig-

*continued*

erate batter in an airtight bowl several hours or overnight.

This will keep for a week or more. To serve, stir batter
thoroughly, and spoon into greased muffin tins, filling
2/3 full. Bake at 400° for 20 minutes or until golden
brown.

**Note:** This batter will double in size, so make sure to
put it in a very large bowl in the refrigerator or you will
have a huge messy surprise later.

*Preparation Time: 15 minutes to make the batter and 3
hours or more refrigeration time*
*Cooking Time: 20 minutes*


## MUSHROOM PÂTÉ

*Makes 8 servings.*
*1 serving or 3 tablespoons = 1 Fat and 1/2 Vegetable
    Exchange.*
*50 calories per serving.*

1/2 cup white wine
3 cloves garlic, chopped
1 onion, chopped
1 pound sliced mushrooms
1/2 teaspoon salt
1/4 teaspoon pepper
8 ounces light cream cheese
1 teaspoon chives

In a large sauté pan sprayed with Pam, bring the white
wine to a boil at high heat. Add garlic and onion. Lower
heat and simmer 5 minutes. Add sliced mushrooms, salt
and pepper; continue to simmer 5 more minutes, or until
mushrooms become browned and pliable. Set aside.

In a food processor or blender, whip cream cheese. Add
sautéed mushroom mixture and chives. Whip until
smooth. Refrigerate several hours before serving. This
will keep a week or may be frozen.

**Note:** I like to eat this as a warm dip. It can also be
used as a pasta sauce if you thin it with evaporated skim
milk, or add crabmeat or salmon, and it is just delicious!

*Preparation Time: 15 minutes to prepare and 2 hours to
refrigerate—can be served imediately.*

# ARTICHOKE CHICKEN

*Makes 4 servings.*
*1 serving or 1 chicken breast = 4 Protein, 2 Vegetable,*
*   and 1/4 Fat Exchange.*
*310 calories per serving.*

4 (4-ounce) chicken breasts
1 (5.5-ounce) can V-8 Juice
3 cloves garlic, crushed
1 small onion
1 (16-ounce) can artichoke hearts, drained and halved
1 (16-ounce) can whole tomatoes, cut into quarters
1 teaspoon basil
2 tablespoons capers (optional)
5 black olives, chopped

In a large sauté pan sprayed with Pam, brown the chicken breasts on both sides. You want to sear the chicken to lock in the juices and brown the exterior. Brown each side approximately 8 minutes and lightly salt and pepper. Lift chicken every few minutes to prevent it from sticking. If it starts to stick, add a small amount of water. When cooked, remove chicken from pan and set aside.

Spray pan again with Pam. Bring the heat to medium/high and add V-8 juice. Add garlic and onion; sauté 5 minutes. Lower heat and add remaining ingredients. Simmer 5 minutes, add chicken, and cover. Cook 25 minutes at a low simmer.

*Preparation Time: 25 minutes*
*Cooking Time: 25 minutes*

Approximately 10% of the calories that you eat are used for digestion. For example, if you eat a muffin that contains 250 calories, your body will expend approximately 25 calories to digest it.

# SPINACH-STRAWBERRY SALAD

*Makes 4 servings.*
*1 serving = 1 Fruit, 2 Vegetable, and 1/2 Fat Exchange.*
*50 calories per serving.*

4 cups spinach, washed and torn
2 cups strawberries, sliced
1/2 cup green onions, sliced
3 tablespoons orange juice
2 tablespoons balsamic vinegar
1 teaspoon olive oil
1 teaspoon chives
1 tablespoon sesame seeds, toasted

Combine spinach, strawberries, and green onion. Set aside. Combine juice, vinegar, oil, and chives; drizzle over the spinach mixture. Sprinkle sesame seeds on top.

*Preparation Time: 10 minutes*

If you want a heart-healthy meal at a fast-food restaurant, choose the grilled chicken sandwich with extra lettuce and tomato, with no mayonnaise or butter on the roll. When eating a salad at a restaurant, ask for your salad dressing on the side.

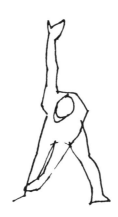

# Low-Fat Diet Plan for Day 30

*Breakfast:*
2 Pumpkin Squares*
1 cup skim milk

*Snack:*
Small banana

*Lunch:*
Large green salad with
2 servings Fresh Peach Salsa*
1 (8-ounce) carton nonfat, sugar-free yogurt

*Dinner:*
2 servings Lasagna (See Index.)
1 ounce toasted Italian bread with Roasted Garlic*
Large green salad with low-calorie dressing

## PUMPKIN SQUARES
*Makes 21 servings.*
*1 serving or 1 pumpkin square = 1 1/3 Bread*
*Exchanges.*
*93 calories per serving.*

4 cups Fiber One Cereal, crushed
2 1/2 cups skim milk
1 large apple, peeled and puréed
20 packets Sweet & Low
2 cups pumpkin (16-ounce can)
2 teaspoons vanilla
1/4 teaspoon nutmeg
1/2 teaspoon cinnamon
1/4 teaspoon ginger
1/4 teaspoon cloves
4 egg whites, beaten
2 cups whole wheat flour
2 tablespoons baking powder
1 teaspoon baking soda
1 teaspoon salt

Crush the Fiber One Cereal in a blender. Pour the 2 1/2 cups milk over the cereal and let stand. In a separate

*continued*

bowl, combine the puréed apple, Sweet & Low, vanilla, spices, and egg whites. Set aside. Mix together the flour, baking powder, baking soda, and salt. Add the Fiber One alternately with the apple mixture to the flour. Mix well. Spray a 13x9-inch baking pan with Pam and pour in the batter. Bake at 350° for 45 minutes. When cooled, cut into 21 squares.

**Note:** These may be made in muffin tins as well. If making muffins, bake at 350° for 25 minutes, or until a toothpick inserted comes out clean.

*Preparation Time: 20 minutes*
*Cooking Time: 45 minutes*


## FRESH PEACH SALSA

*Makes 10 servings.*
*1 serving = 1 Fruit Exchange.*
*40 calories per serving.*

10 peaches, peeled and diced
1/4 cup red onion, diced
2 tablespoons cilantro
2 tablespoons rice vinegar
1 teaspoon lemon juice
1 clove garlic, minced

Combine all ingredients in a bowl, stirring well. Cover and refrigerate.

**Note:** This is great to serve with chicken!

*Preparation Time: 10 minutes*

 Spread your food intake throughout the day to keep your metabolism going.

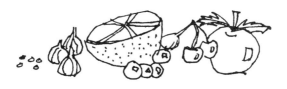

# ROASTED GARLIC

*Unlimited vegetable.*
*Pig out and enjoy!*

**1 head garlic**
**1 teaspoon water**

Remove the outermost leaves of the garlic. Cut the top off of the garlic head, exposing the garlic inside. Wrap the garlic in aluminum foil, sprinkling the water on top of the exposed garlic before sealing. Bake at 325° for 1 hour. When garlic is baked, squeeze out the garlic paste and spread on bread, crackers or whatever you want!

**Note:** I roast a dozen heads at a time and squeeze out the paste into an airtight container. I use this in place of regular garlic in all of my recipes for a special zip! This is great whipped together with cottage cheese and spread on a bagel for lunch!!

 Every calorie counts, so "invest" them wisely.

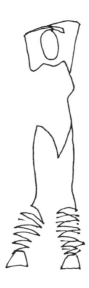

# INDEX

Cynthia Martino presents seminars on nutrition, exercise, and weight loss throughout the Atlanta region. Additionally, she enjoys teaching low-fat cooking classes, creating delicious, savory meals that are kind to the waistline.

If you are interested in having Mrs. Martino as a guest lecturer, or for cooking demonstrations, please contact Quail Ridge Press as 1-800-343-1583.

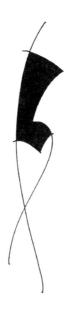

## "Best of the Best" Cookbook Series:

| | | | | | |
|---|---|---|---|---|---|
| *Alabama* | (28-3) $14.95 | | *New England* | (50-X) | $16.95 |
| *Arkansas* | (43-7) $14.95 | | *North Carolina* | (38-0) | $14.95 |
| *Florida* | (16-X) $14.95 | | *Ohio* | (68-2) | $14.95 |
| *Georgia* | (30-5) $14.95 | | *Oklahoma* | (65-8) | $14.95 |
| *Illinois* | (58-5) $14.95 | | *Pennsylvania* | (47-X) | $14.95 |
| *Indiana* | (57-7) $14.95 | | *South Carolina* | (39-9) | $14.95 |
| *Kentucky* | (27-5) $14.95 | | *Tennessee* | (20-8) | $14.95 |
| *Louisiana* | (13-5) $14.95 | | *Texas* | (14-3) | $14.95 |
| *Michigan* | (69-0) $14.95 | | *Texas II* | (62-3) | $16.95 |
| *Mississippi* | (19-4) $14.95 | | *Virginia* | (41-0) | $14.95 |
| *Missouri* | (44-5) $14.95 | | | | |

Individuals may purchase this 21-volume set for a special "Best Club" price of $230.00 (a 28% discount off the regular price) plus $6.00 shipping. Becoming a member of the "Best Club" will entitle you to a 25% discount on future volumes.

## Other Quail Ridge Press Cookbooks:

| | ISBN Suffix |
|---|---|
| *The Little New Orleans Cookbook* (h/b) $8.95 | 42-9 |
| *The Little New Orleans Cookbook (French)* $10.95 | 60-7 |
| *The Little Gumbo Book* (hardbound) $8.95 | 17-8 |
| *The Little Bean Book* (hardbound) $9.95 | 32-1 |
| *The Complete Venison Cookbook* $16.95 (p/b) | 70-4 |
| *Eat Your Way Thin* $9.95 | 76-3 |
| *Gourmet Camping* $9.95 | 45-3 |
| *Lite Up Your Life* $14.95 | 40-2 |
| *Hors D'Oeuvres Everybody Loves* $5.95 | 11-9 |
| *The Seven Chocolate Sins* $5.95 | 01-1 |
| *A Salad A Day* $5.95 | 02-X |
| *Quickies for Singles* $5.95 | 03-8 |
| *The Twelve Days of Christmas Cookbook* $5.95 | 00-3 |
| *The Country Mouse Cheese Cookbook* $5.95 | 10-0 |

ISBN Prefix: 0-937552-. All books are comb bound unless noted otherwise. Prices subject to change. To order by mail, send check or money order to:

## QUAIL RIDGE PRESS
### P. O. Box 123 / Brandon, MS 39043

Or call toll-free to order by credit card:
### 1-800-343-1583

Please add $2.00 postage for any amount of books sent to one address. Gift wrap with enclosed card add $1.50. Mississipp residents add 7% sales tax. Write or call for free brochure of all QRP books.